Cheap Talk

Corporealities: Discourses of Disability

Series editors: David T. Mitchell and Sharon L. Snyder

Recent Titles

Cheap Talk: Disability and the Politics of Communication
by Joshua St. Pierre

Diaphanous Bodies: Ability, Disability, and Modernist Irish Literature
by Jeremy Colangelo

Embodied Archive: Disability in Post-Revolutionary Mexican Cultural Production
by Susan Antebi

Beholding Disability in Renaissance England
by Allison P. Hobgood

A History of Disability, New Edition
by Henri-Jacques Stiker

Vitality Politics: Health, Debility, and the Limits of Black Emancipation
by Stephen Knadler

Blindness Through the Looking Glass: The Performance of Blindness, Gender, and the Sensory Body
by Gili Hammer

HandiLand: The Crippest Place on Earth
by Elizabeth A. Wheeler

The Matter of Disability: Materiality, Biopolitics, Crip Affect
by David T. Mitchell, Susan Antebi, and Sharon L. Snyder, editors

Monstrous Kinds: Body, Space, and Narrative in Renaissance Representations of Disability
by Elizabeth B. Bearden

Autistic Disturbances: Theorizing Autism Poetics from the DSM *to* Robinson Crusoe
by Julia Miele Rodas

Foucault and Feminist Philosophy of Disability
by Shelley L. Tremain

Academic Ableism: Disability and Higher Education
by Jay Timothy Dolmage

Negotiating Disability: Disclosure and Higher Education
by Stephanie L. Kerschbaum, Laura T. Eisenman, and James M. Jones, editors

Portraits of Violence: War and the Aesthetics of Disfigurement
by Suzannah Biernoff

Bodies of Modernism: Physical Disability in Transatlantic Modernist Literature
by Maren Tova Linett

War on Autism: On the Cultural Logic of Normative Violence
by Anne McGuire

The Biopolitics of Disability: Neoliberalism, Ablenationalism, and Peripheral Embodiment
by David T. Mitchell with Sharon L. Snyder

Foucault and the Government of Disability, Enlarged and Revised Edition
by Shelley Tremain, editor

A complete list of titles in the series can be found at www.press.umich.edu

Cheap Talk

Disability and the Politics of Communication

Joshua St. Pierre

University of Michigan Press
Ann Arbor

Published in the United States of America by the
University of Michigan Press
Printed and bound by CPI Group (UK) Ltd, Croydon, CR0 4YY

First published May 2022

A CIP catalog record for this book is available from the British Library.

Library of Congress Cataloging-in-Publication data has been applied for.

ISBN 978-0-472-07534-8 (hardcover: alk. paper)
ISBN 978-0-472-05534-0 (paper: alk. paper)
ISBN 978-0-472-22014-4 (e-book)

This research was undertaken, in part, thanks to funding from the
Canada Research Chairs Program.

Cover description: The background of the cover is taken up by a large graphic of a blue megaphone. The words "Cheap Talk" are in white letters, with "Disability and the Politics of Communication" in light blue letters just below. "Joshua St. Pierre" appears in white letters at the bottom of the cover.

For Charis, through thick and thin.

Contents

Digital materials related to this title can be found on the Fulcrum platform via the following citable URL: https://doi.org/10.3998/mpub.12158924

Acknowledgments

This book is the product of many voices, and it would be a mistake to ascribe it to a single author. Words from Octavia Butler (1993, 3) come to mind—"All that you touch, you change. All that you change, changes you"—and I am full of gratitude for the many people who have changed me and this project over the past eight years. *Cheap Talk* took root when I was a PhD student in the Department of Philosophy at the University of Alberta. Cressida Heyes is—sorry, literally everyone else—the best supervisor in the business. She not only supported my weird hunches and dysfluent process, welcomed me into a feminist community, and helped give me a career, she modelled a fierce intellectual life abundant with grace and mirth. I am also thankful for the many brilliant mentors and colleagues from the University of Alberta who, in many different ways, have supported me and this project, including Catherine Kellogg, Rob Aitken, Robert Nichols, Rob Wilson, Marie-Eve Morin, Catherine Clune-Taylor, Jana Smith Elford, Emily Douglas, Megan Dean, Esther Rosario, Felicity Bohnet, and especially Kristin Rodier.

I am grateful beyond words for my found family: the disability studies and activism community. This project is the result of many long and generous conversations. I have presented various early drafts of this project to the Canadian Disability Studies Association, the Society for Disability Studies, and the Canadian Society for Women in Philosophy, and this book has been deeply shaped in these communities of practice. I am especially thankful for Jay Dolmage, for his mentorship and for modelling critical disability scholarship done right. He has also encouraged and supported this project at every halting step. Danielle Peers, Ada Jaarsma, Robert McRuer, Emily Anne Parker, Kelly Fritsch, and Anne McGuire have all offered insightful feedback on (sometimes proto) sections of this project, and I have been enriched by engaging with their ideas in the process of writing and rewriting. The voices of so many in the stuttering community are also in this book. I am indebted especially to Zara Richter and Erin Schick, and to those within the "Metaphoric Stammers and Embodied Speakers" network who are growing our little subfield of dysfluency studies. I am lucky to have interlocutors such as Maria Stuart, Daniel Martin, Chris Eagle, Roshaya Rodness, JJJJJerome Ellis, Patrick Campbell, Chris Constantino, and Sam Simpson.

This book was still in rough shape when I taught it as a seminar, and I am thankful for the patience of the brilliant group of students in POLS 410 (Winter 2020) who helped me piece the project together, especially Ronald Espiritu, Celina Gado, Alexandria Hammond, Joshua Beatty, Emily Proskiw, and Ben Sugars. This book would still be a mess without the incredible work of Rissa Reist, Luke Sandle, and Dani Jorgenson as my RAs this past year. Dani went above and beyond and was essential in getting this book over the finish line. I must owe her coffee for life.

My thanks to Sara Cohen at University of Michigan Press, who has been so supportive of this project, and also to the two anonymous reviewers who offered generous comments and much to think about.

Many dear friends have given their time to read drafts or offer other support when life was difficult. I am especially thankful for Jessie Beier, Dan Gabor, Joel From, Rebecca Tait, Brady Van Leenan, Matt Johnson, Kimberly Williams, Tyler Williams, Amber Bergsma, and Phil Bergsma.

What would I have done without my mother-in-law, Grace Banks? Our many walks and conversations have brought this project into focus. It may be, as I argue in this book, that many truths are unspeakable. But for everything else, I'm glad the world has her.

Finally, Charis. I find myself already in the ineffable, for there are no words for my gratitude and devotion to you that don't turn cheap on my tongue. Thank you for our little life forged together in fear and trembling.

A section of chapter 1 was published in an earlier version as Joshua St. Pierre and Charis St. Pierre, "Governing the Voice: A Critical History of Speech-Language Pathology," *Foucault Studies* 24 (2018): 151–84. Chapter 4 was published in an earlier version as "Talking Heads and Shitting in the Street: Stuttering Parrhesia in Three Modes," *Journal of Interdisciplinary Voice Studies* 5, no. 2 (2020): 179–95. https://doi.org/10.1386/jivs_00024_1

Preface

Four notes.

One. I admit (and enjoy) the irony of a stutterer spinning over 60,000 words about cheap talk. The book would be better, and probably more truthful, as an audiobook stuttered aloud, but do we have that kind of time?

Two. I try to avoid feeding voices that suck all the oxygen out of the room and render us unable to discuss anything else. Thus, for the most part, I intentionally do not name prominent trolls and talking heads in this book—I leave such pragmatic connections to the reader.

Three. It is this same longing for oxygen that stays my hand from the obvious Deleuzian reading of "stuttering" that tracks clichés about dysfluency all over good theory. While Deleuze is one interlocutor in this book, I am far more interested in rough ground than smooth paths. I agree with Foucault (1980, 53–54) that "[t]he only valid tribute to thought such as Nietzsche's [or Foucault's, Deleuze's, . . .] is precisely to use it, to deform it, to make it groan and protest" in large part because this approach to theory hews closer to lived experience.

Four. I should warn readers hoping for solutions or cures for cheap talk that this book will probably be a great disappointment for you. I don't believe there are "fixes" for this mess, especially not universal ones. The best I hope is that this book might offer a pragmatic that changes, in nitty-gritty ways, how we communicate: how we look (or don't look) at nonnormative speakers, how we listen, how we speak, how our bodies respond to difference. I don't claim this book to be parrhesiastic in the slightest, but I do believe that listening more carefully to the groans of bodies in communication can invite new becomings.

Introduction

Stuttering, Trolls, and Talking Heads

The Soviets used to say that the United States had free speech
but no one could hear you over the noise of machines.
Today no one can hear you over the noise of talk.
—Fred Moten and Stefano Harney

Communication has always underwhelmed me. The dream that more information and less noise will produce a better world (a common dream even in progressive circles) is hard to take seriously for those who struggle to not-be-noise on a daily basis. But the cultural wisdom, the axiom, if you want, is that more information and better communication will help us avoid errors and cultivate responsible action. Given enough talk, given enough data, we might understand the Other and resolve conflict—from the intrapersonal, to the intersubjective, to the international, and even on the ecological scale. Perfect communication is, of course, a myth, yet one that can be profoundly productive. Who would stand against more and better communication? And who, not incidentally, can be heard over all the noise of talk?

I began this project in 2016, writing on the politics and production of disabled speech. I was interested in the challenges of speaking while disabled in a world saturated by "cheap talk"—a common phrase I stretch to mean speech disconnected from action as well as speech rendered as a cheap resource of connectivity. As chance would have it, I found myself undertaking this work surrounded by the overwhelming clatter of populist movements such as Brexit and MAGA, perfect examples of Gilles Deleuze's (1990, 175) insistence that speech and communication have become corrupted and permeated by money, and thus, by extension, that "[w]e don't suffer these days from any lack of communication, but rather from all the forces making us say things when we've nothing much to say" (137). My digital and social spaces were increasingly bombarded with political opinions, banter, bullshit, and memes. But what struck me most about the mechanisms of cheap talk, those "forces that make us say things when we've nothing much to say," is that they implicate not just the talking head on cable news, and not just the online troll spreading misinformation, but also my own stuttered voice.

By that time, I had spent decades attempting to liberate my voice from the restraints of disability through a host of therapeutic technologies so that my true, *fluent*, voice could "be heard." This practice is common for disabled speakers. After all, the clerics of the information age, from speech-language pathologists to Silicon Valley CEOs, all construe dysfluent communication as an impediment to full humanness and render perfect meaning and smooth and instant connection, what I will call fluency, an unassailable good. Acting as a prerequisite for dysfluent speakers to "be heard" as full social and political beings, the imperative of therapeutic intervention on the body is another instrument of cheap talk.

Cheap Talk argues that neoliberalism makes fluent communication an unquestionable good by first rendering communication a distinctly *technical* rather than political event: not a shared navigation across difference, but the exchange of information by "equal" agents in a decontextualised matrix. Since neoliberalism is the stage for much of this book, it deserves some early introduction. Put generally, neoliberalism is a political economic project that, since the '70s, has worked to liberate the market, especially finance capital, from internal and external constraints and to reorganise society according to the logic and needs of the market. David Harvey (2007, 2) explains that in one regard, neoliberalism "proposes that human well-being can best be advanced by liberating individual entrepreneurial freedoms and skills within an institutional framework characterized by strong private property rights, free markets, and free trade." With the help of information and communication technologies that untether us from traditional boundaries of time and space, neoliberalism "frees" individuals to be their own enterprises and to thus take charge of themselves, now unburdened by the rigidity of the "nanny state" and demand-side economics.

Disability theorists Anne McGuire and Kelly Fritsch (2019, 91) accordingly describe the contemporary neoliberal subject as a "productive, competitive, entrepreneurial, freelance, flexible subject, who labours continuously to optimize herself, thereby ensuring her value as human capital." McGuire and Fritsch alert us to the fact that if human betterment is the neoliberal carrot, the brutal logic of the market is the stick. The neoliberal state divests its responsibility to produce and repair human capital, while at the same time creating the conditions for hypercompetition and social inequality (Brown 2015, 42). Thus, the neoliberal subject is cut from the social contract and made responsible for its individual survival: to gain a competitive advantage, to increase one's brand rating, to see a return on investment in human capital. Submitting to a host of purportedly neutral therapeutic interventions on the self is central to the process. From the perspective of this book, neoliberalism is a hostile terrain not merely because it marketises all domains of life, but more fully, as Jay Dolmage (2016, 111) argues, because it is a "system that powerfully *masks* inequalities and readily *co-opts* concepts such as autonomy, diversity, tolerance, and democracy" (emphases mine). It turns out that masking inequality and co-opting democratic values are also two functions of cheap talk.

The political character of talk has been assaulted under neoliberal policies and practices. In its colloquial usage, the phrase "talk is cheap" refers to questions of political action. Cheap talk is that which is uncoupled from both action and truth. The vast but empty promises of political candidates come first to mind, but we might also consider the devil's advocate, the middle manager, the shock jock, the internet troll. Cheap talk is a positive feedback loop that spreads, speech freed from regulation to spin on wheels of infinite production. And here emerges the second, economic, meaning of cheap talk. As I will argue throughout, cheap talk is that that is *made cheap* and rendered via a stable, low-cost, and reliable resource stream. Neoliberalism formats and activates the powers of communication held in the individual and social body according to the specific needs of capital. These two mutually dependent valences of cheap talk, political and economic, incite and reinforce each other in complex ways.

Cheap talk courses through everyday life. For example, while content users across the political spectrum may share and debate the same news article on social media with either outrage or admiration, content *producers* operate within a fundamentally different economy: not one of truth, but of clicks. As comedian Michelle Wolf (2018) remarks, "a share is a share is a share is a share." To take another example, cheap talk keeps corporate wheels in motion. Writer Anna Wiener (2020) calls the jargon-y language of corporate spaces "garbage language." These are vacuous sentences filled with words such as "optionality" or "deliverables" that have a "scammy flavour" (Young 2020) and that mystify underlings and deflect responsibility away from the managerial class. "The hideous nature of these words—their facility to warp and impede communication—is also their purpose" (Young 2020). Cheap talk is everywhere and its functions are legion. As I will argue in chapter 3, blocking access to privileged flows of knowledge while masking these inequalities is chief among the functions of cheap talk. In itself, passing along a cliché is hardly negative. For instance, Martin Heidegger (1962, 172) describes speech that circulates a familiar stock of words and ideas as "idle talk," a term that sounds pejorative but is for Heidegger the ground from which meaningful talk can emerge. But while cheap and idle talk share a family resemblance, what distinguishes cheap talk, as the example above demonstrates, are techniques that mobilise and weaponise pointless statements for neoliberal ends. I suggest that an analysis of the relations between the stutterer, troll, and talking head can provide an inroad to the concept of cheap talk. Allow me to clear some conceptual space with two vignettes.

Vignette 1: Talking Heads, Interrupted

In March 2017, Robert Kelly, an academic living in Seoul, went viral when his BBC interview was interrupted by two children who burst through the unlocked door into the live frame. Fifteen seconds later, a panicked woman rushes to herd the children—now tugging at the talking head—out of the room. The interview closes with embarrassed smiles. "We both assumed that was the end of my career as a talking head," Kelly and his wife said later (Usborne 2017). Why? Because talking heads are cheap and easily replaced. Because the talking head is a fragile nexus of information and affect ruined by even mundane interruptions. Nevertheless, this particular mutation happened to go viral, invoking both delight and criticism around the globe.

Interruptions reveal hidden processes and differentials—here, how a talking head gets made. Like all products of capital, the talking head is a fetishisation; the "expert knower," a seemingly mystical object that hides its constitutive social and material relations. In this case, feminists on social media were quick to point out the gendered labour hidden very literally behind closed doors. Such invisible labour supports and makes the talking head possible. Put otherwise, the talking head is always produced within a *clearing*—of space, of time, of noise, of interrelation—and requires such a sterile environment to maintain the fiction of frictionless and automatic connection.

Vignette 2: The Troll

At 55 Savushkina Street, St. Petersburg, a Kremlin-backed "troll farm" runs shifts of paid trolls to carry out misinformation strategies around the globe. "Each worker," explains Lyudmila Savchuk, the Russian activist who first broke the story in 2014, "has a quota to fill every day and every night. Because the factory works around the clock. It never stops. Not for a second" (Maynes 2019). The return on investment is quite remarkable. These are the soldiers of the new psychological warfare who carry inexpensive memes and bullshit into battle; Russia is but one actor in this information frontier. In general, the troll is one who assumes a false online identity to sow intentional discord with inflammatory and misleading comments. Some troll for pure amusement, others are more strategic. In addition to the troll farms, we might, for example, consider prominent UK politicians who campaigned for Brexit with silver tongues making great promises *up until the very moment they won*, at which point they promptly disavowed each pledge they had made. Politics has become an art of trolling the polity with cheap talk. Sophistry is of course an ancient practice—said Gorgias to Socrates (1994, 24), "Rhetoric is the only area of expertise you need to learn. You can ignore all the rest and still get the better of the professionals!"—yet perhaps trolling divorces speech from truth once and for all.

Trolls are what Harry Frankfurt (2005, 30) calls "bullshitters" who deliberately misrepresent, yet don't precisely *lie* insofar as lying implies a continued commitment to truth (by negation). The bullshitter, the troll, on the other hand, makes statements that are thoroughly "unconnected to a concern with truth." It is such that the troll argues in bad faith; any statement is a lure that, when pressed, will collapse upon itself with a smirk. Trolls, as Sartre (1948, 13) already noted of the anti-Semite, "seek not to persuade by sound argument but to intimidate and disconcert."

• • •

At face value, the troll and talking head are different creatures. The talking head descends from the line of priests; the troll from scoundrels. Dan Nimmo and James Combs (1992, 35) insist that pundits wield authority via their secret knowledge (of how the world *really* is), which is confirmed onscreen with "striking appearances or styles to complement priestly words spoken with an inspiring voice." They note that over the twentieth century, as more informational priests crowded the field, each claiming to speak truth above the noise, each vying for their share of collective attention, the role of the talking head has pluralised: from sober priest to entertainer, demagogue, and therapist. But consistent is the capacity to connect audiences through feedback loops of attention, affect, and capital. "The more quotable the talking priestly head, the more authority the pundit has; the more authority, the more request for sound bites" (45). The more powerful the outburst of the talking head, the more capacity to generate affective resonance, the more shareable the link. From cable news to YouTube personalities, the talking head now dominates our screens. It is a *thing* aptly named: ripped from the body and reterritorialised on the stage of signification and capital.

The troll, on the other hand, has thrived not in informational temples and highways, but under its bridges, in its cellars and labyrinth passages. It is true that some trolls have gone mainstream, replacing the authority that comes with anonymity with the authority of a face. As Sarah Sharma (2020, 172) quips, "We are faced with the onslaught of trolls and peons who have turned into pundits and presidents by way of access to Wi-Fi." Going mainstream rapidly alters the habitat of such trolls: as they become talking heads, they enter the homogenising economy of clicks and attention. But the troll nevertheless still often prefers anonymity—provoking and manipulating in the dark, distrusting and refusing to engage with the pundits, academics, and scientists who represent the elite establishment. In this regard trolls are kin to representatives of the trickster archetype, such as Hermes, the Jackal, or Coyote. The trickster, as Whitney Phillips (2015, 9) explains, is "[b]oth culture-hero and culture-villain. He—and tricksters are almost always gendered male—invents lies to preserve the truth." Phillips notes that the troll similarly claims an amoral position; neither good nor evil, trolls speak chaos to power (although often at the expense of distinctions such as punching up vs. down).

But despite their many differences, the troll and talking head are kin, the former an alter ego of the latter. Trolls and talking heads are what we get when communication functions increasingly as capital. Both leverage and seek to materialise the hypermobility and speed of neoliberal capital. To draw value from communication, info-capitalism must render it cheap and relatively predictable. However, it does not simply "tame" the embodied powers of communication to make them flow in reliable channels, but rather it metastasises communication itself, making the *desire* for maximal and automatic connection internal to its machineries of accumulation. It is such that the talking head and troll represent two modes of cheapening talk, two sides of the same coin. I turn now to consider how the voice of the dysfluent speaker resonates with both.

The talking head epitomises the commodification of speech. It is a connection machine that spews soundbites to keep the flow of information and affect in resonant circulation. In this regard, the talking head manifests a particular process of becoming-machine and becoming-human capital. Those with dysfluent speech often yearn to become talking heads to avoid stigma and even to "be heard" as social and political agents. Yet once reduced to a talking head, one can at best aspire to be a soundbite. And if "finding one's voice" or "speaking out" are problematic for *any* citizen, what then of those of us (disabled and marginalised peoples) who make such deplorable talking heads? Yes, therapeutic technologies can sometimes rehabilitate disabled voices. And yes, disabled people make excellent *props* that—when staged and edited right—can evoke powerful affect. But try to stutter truth-to-power outside the assigned lane of pity, inspiration, authenticity, identity, or even equality? My voice can't keep pace with normative registers of time and resolves once again to noise. My face stutters, the talking head morphs and becomes grotesque—now *draining* attention and capital. Cut to commercial.

The troll presents its own dangers. That trolls "seek not to persuade by sound argument but to intimidate and disconcert" suggests a turn from a humanist logic of persuasion towards a logic of the machine. Trolls overwhelm with information and affect (anger, fear) rather than seeking to persuade or compel with sound argument, and can, in this way, operate akin to denial-of-service cyberattacks that flood a system with repeated requests, overloading it and shutting it down. The troll (whether tweeting from St. Petersburg or the White House) hacks and confuses the human psyche with the inhuman *speed* by which it can flit from one bullshit talking point to another. RAND Corporation (an American think tank) has labelled this the "firehose of falsehood"—a new model of propaganda that is "rapid, continuous, and repetitive, [and] lacks commitment to consistency" (Paul and Matthews 2016, 16). The troll seeks not, at least directly, to replace one ideology with another (one signal for another), but to increase the ratio of noise to signal, making the very effort to differentiate signal from noise or lie from truth impossible and ultimately comedic. The production of this type of uncertainty is often intentional.

For the troll, language cannot be taken too seriously within a digital semiotic environment of near infinite circulation (e.g., retweets, memes, copypasta). If you will allow me some editorial freedom, Sartre is again instructive. For while he is writing about the anti-Semite, not the troll, I suggest we can find resonance between these figures:

> [A]t the outset he has chosen to devaluate words and reasons. How entirely at ease he feels as a result. . . . [Trolls] know that their remarks are frivolous, open to challenge. But they are amusing themselves, for it is their adversary who is obliged to use words responsibly, since he believes in words. The [trolls] have the right to play. (13)

At first glance the disabled speaker and troll have little in common. One struggles to emit speech, struggles to be heard, and struggles to be taken seriously; the other spews information like a machine and, at some level, must not be found to be *too* serious. And while the troll deals in a seemingly infinite economy, ours is finite (it takes effort to communicate, so we often choose words with care). Yet the troll and the dysfluent are nevertheless strange bedfellows—agents of disconnection—that raise troubling questions around political action. Paul Virilio (1999, 141) writes that in the (now arrived) information war, "it will be entirely impossible to distinguish a deliberate action from an involuntary reaction or an 'accident'; or to distinguish an attack from a mere technical breakdown." Within information societies, can the deliberate, machinic attack of the troll be differentiated from the involuntary "technical breakdown" of the stutter? Are information attacks or breakdowns the only options available to the disabled rhetor?

To gain traction on these questions, this book builds towards and concludes with an examination of the contemporary conditions of truth-telling. Thinking with both Gilles Deleuze and Michel Foucault, I suggest that reducing communication to the logic and value of the market—epitomised in the expression "the marketplace of ideas"—has produced what Foucault (2001) anticipated as a "*parrhesiastic* crisis," that is, a crisis of truth-telling, that washes away the conditions for speaking truth to power in a sea of equality. The marketplace of ideas renders us ostensibly equal talking heads, yet equality is always a necessary yet not sufficient condition for rising to speak against power. Foucault argues that the *parrhesiastes* forms an "ethical differentiation" or specific self-relation (one, for example, of courage). I argue it is this capacity for self-positioning that neoliberalism seeks to neutralise such that the enunciation can only draw on *formal* right and equality in a hollow expression of "free speech" paraded endlessly in social media. It is here that a critical attention to the materiality of dysfluent speech can help us reconsider the agency of communication.

Cheap Info

Allow me to re-approach the concept of cheap talk from a different angle. It is easy to be fooled by the hyperpartisan flourish of trolls and talking heads, so I want to be clear: the production of cheap talk relies everywhere on the depoliticisation of communication. Cheap talk, put otherwise, displaces a shared traversal of difference with a technocratic exchange of messages. A capture of communicability lies at the heart of this reduction. Historian and sociologist Jason Moore (2015) argues that we should not read capitalism through a narrow economic lens of wage-labour, but understand it as a planetary-historical system that must continually appropriate *extra*-economic zones of life. It is this appropriation that makes the wage-labour relation conceptually and materially possible. As he writes: "Capital must not only ceaselessly accumulate and revolutionize commodity production; it must ceaselessly search for, and find ways to produce, Cheap Natures: a rising stream of low-cost food, labor-power, energy, and raw materials" (53). Put otherwise: resource streams must be *made* cheap for the law of capitalist value to hold. The production of Cheap Natures such as Food, Oil, and Housework is the engine of industrial capitalism. But following the shift from industrial to postindustrial capitalism (what I am calling "info-capitalism"), I believe it necessary to consider also the production of "Cheap Information." Info-capitalism survives only through its hunt for and production of low-cost information. It persists through the continual appropriation of untapped wells of communicability constituted and exploited through the body.

We should note that Cheap Info would straddle several of Moore's categories. It is, yes, an extension of labour-power, but also a raw material for info-capitalism and a peculiar type of fixed capital. Ursula Huws (2014), a theorist of labour, argues that the nineteenth-century desire for a literate and articulate population was in part a bourgeois strategy to deflate the bargaining power of the surging workforce of clerks needed in the global trade industry. Yet the concept of "information" and thus of Cheap Info extends beyond the domain of labour and the subject. It refers more fully to the *encoded flow of a message* between any sender and receiver—human or not. For instance, today it is algorithms that trade most stocks worldwide: machines talk to machines, and humans are mere attendants. In this way, the contemporary is "machinic"—largely populated and run not by individuals and representations, but by the collective assemblages of bodies and signs that constitute inhuman life, such as algorithms, viral talking heads, ghostly call centre voices, deep fakes, or online trolls.

The liberal apologist might interrupt to proclaim the benefits of finding new territories to mine for Cheap Info. Incarnate in the body politic, Cheap Info facilitates knowledge, expression, and dialogue—the lifeblood of liberal democracies. And the neoliberal will of course insist that we need Cheap Info to guarantee equal opportunity in the social, political, and economic market. More specifically, procuring a steady flow of Cheap Info is a prerequisite for attaining a state of "perfect information," a term that describes an ideal state where each market actor (consumer and producer alike) possesses complete knowledge of past and present events. Market signals (prices) express such vast flows of information that the State, let alone the individual, cannot hope to process and act accordingly. Yes, the market is a "rising tide [that] lifts all boats" from poverty and human misery (Harvey 2007, 64), but this promise is conditional and will materialise only after we feed the market *sufficient information* to manage the future and thus only when information, like capital, is allowed to flow unfettered by regulation and boundaries of any kind.

Thus does late liberalism govern the flow of information across material bodies with a panoply of therapeutic techniques. And thus does it recode this flow of Cheap Info, cheap talk, as a pre-eminent social and even moral good. We now *must* circulate information to stay informed and connected, we *must* speak with others to be productive, we *must* communicate to be understood, well-adjusted, and happy. "Communication" stands in for liberal-democratic ideals of understanding, tolerance, inclusion, and deliberation. It facilitates "free" expression; it negotiates and resolves alterity; it sustains social cohesion. "Technical networks," writes historian of information Ronald Day (2001, 74), "are not in themselves socially communicative, but as social tropes they have the power to construct—not only technically but also socially—a future based on a vision of social connectivity and communication." Who would oppose this future of Cheap Info? Who would take the side of misunderstanding, breakdown, and disconnection?

Such questions are of course meant to silence discussion, but they could just as easily be points of departure. Drawing attention to cheap talk, to those forces that incite the proliferation of communication only to detach it from its sources, is a central object of this book because it flips the politics of communication ability and disability. On one hand, it reveals that fluency is not a natural condition, but one that must be maintained through ongoing biopolitical investments. And from the other side, if, as Deleuze (1990, 129) writes, "[w]hat we're plagued by these days isn't any blocking of communication, but pointless statements," then disability, an ostensible blockage of information and affect, might represent not diminished agency but a critical opening in systems of power. In other words, what if the communicative flood in which we participate daily is hardly a utopia of free expression, but is rather a type of priestly service to and for the machines? Fluent speech is premised on the mythic conception of an individual free utterance that the dysfluent tongue or the neurodivergent brain impedes, such that exposing the normative dimensions of communication societies fundamentally recasts the "problem" of communication disability.

A Primer on Fluency

I engage many interlocuters in this critique of cheap talk, from disciplines including political theory, feminist theory, and communication studies, but situate myself within the field of critical disability studies (CDS) and the burgeoning subfield of dysfluency studies (cf. St. Pierre 2012; Eagle 2013; Martin and Stuart 2021). One of the main contributions I seek to make in this book, a contribution CDS enables, is to disrupt the presumed smoothness of info-capitalism by placing the unruly and fragile body at the centre of analysis.

The field of CDS contests the premise that disability is a simple biological fact and demonstrates that what we call "disability" is a complex interaction between corporeality and social, discursive, and material processes—a "social and political category of difference" (Erevelles 2011, 2). The binaries of normal/abnormal and abled/disabled are historically specific means of managing populations. This point is made well by Shelley Tremain (2001, 632), who argues that biological differences are "materialized as universal attributes (properties) of subjects through the iteration and reiteration of rather culturally specific regulatory norms and ideals about (for example) human function and structure, competency, intelligence, and ability." But much like feminist theory, I understand CDS to be a set of methodological commitments rather than a circumscribed object of study. CDS obviously involves the study of disability, just as feminist theory interrogates sex and gender. Yet more than a discourse about disability, CDS is also a jumping-off point to *do theory*. What happens, in other words, if we take the dysfluent subject rather than the hyperfluent subject as our starting point for analysing rhetoric, politics, or power? What thinking is made possible by starting from material experiences of disability and disability relations?

This book is thus about fluency—about the connections that it relies on, that it opens up, and that it forecloses. In the context of disability, "fluency" refers to the process of speaking smoothly, without stutters, ticks, repetitions, slurs, blocks, etc. In general, I understand fluency to be an assembly of forces that seeks to make information flow unchecked across material bodies. Fluency is what Foucault calls a *dispositif*—a congealing of power and knowledge in the flesh of communicative bodies. Yet it is also a critical lens through which political action can be appraised and reimagined. Foucault insists (1984, 343) "not that everything is bad, but that everything is dangerous." Likewise, I seek to map both the possibilities and dangers of the ideal of perfect meaning and its incarnation (or rather, approximation in flesh).

Within the cultural imaginary, we often fantasise that normalised, fluent speech constitutes what fluid mechanists call a "laminar flow." This term describes a perfectly smooth and thus transparent current that passes without resistance or repetition—without turbulence, water appears not to move at all! A dysfluent phenomenon such as a stutter is contrarily a *thing* that obstructs the normal flow of communicability to produce both eddies and zones of stagnancy in its wake. The eddy describes a void into which water rushes upstream and holds flotsam in its power for an undetermined time until it spits something out. The stutter introduces vortices into a smooth flow and thus renders communication nontransparent. Will the dysfluent message arrive, or will it be caught in cycles of repetition? What are they thinking? *Can* they think? *Can this subject even conduct a current?* The fear of the stutter as a deathly repetition is ubiquitous, not just in culture, but in everyday life. Will this awkward conversation with a stutterer never end? Will the stutter of this potential employee sink my business? Will this student's repetitions take up too much classroom space? Will these delays impede their classmates? Will the dysfluent adult who lives in shame finally leave the house today?

To consider fluency in terms of fluid dynamics is to stretch its meaning, but only slightly. The most common definition of fluency, though the least related to my project, involves a familiarity within a cultural world: "I speak English fluently." This notion of fluency depicts one's familiarity with a language and, as Maria Lugones (1987) argues, the way we *move* or "travel" within and across such worlds. The connection with fluid dynamics is even more clear in the second, medical-therapeutic, definition of fluency: "I went to speech therapy because my speech is *not* fluent." In his well-used textbook on speech disabilities, Barry Guitar (2006, 13), a speech-language pathologist, offers an exemplary definition: "simply . . . the effortless flow of speech." This is offered in the midst of caveats and backtracking. Guitar readily admits (12) that fluency is difficult to pin down and that researchers within speech-language pathology often focus on what it is not—namely, dysfluency. Here are a few characteristics of fluency, according to the so-called experts of the voice: a lack of hesitation, the "rhythmical" patterning that follows a normalised cadence, the lack of "extra sounds." Fluency is defined by the overall rate of speech, which includes not just the rate of vocal flow but of *information* flow (Starkweather 1987); by the clarity of meaning; and lastly, by a lack of "effort" on the part of the speaker. Together, the medical-therapeutic definition describes speech that is perfectly smooth, mastered, and transparent like a laminar flow.

To think about fluency in terms of flow is also to think about junctions: how are flows maintained in their connections and disconnections? In chapter 3 I develop a concept of "machinic fluency" that describes the functional capacity to interface with other component parts of an information system. To be fluent in this sense is to be *a smooth site of contact* that is universally connectible. The machinic tongue—the instrument of talking head and troll alike—can exchange information quickly and efficiently with nearly any other component part (human or not). Fluency is thus not simply the demand for intelligibility and understanding produced on the social stage. It is machinic: an imperative to communicate as the machine, to maximise our communicative inputs and outputs, to optimise our connectivity.

The machinic tongue overcodes political action. Jodi Dean (2009) describes our contemporary political state as "communicative capitalism," where participation within flows of information offers the appearance of political action. Even though such communicative fields are constituted by the exchange of messages, it is their circulation through smooth contact, rather than their representational content and subjective uptake, that stands at centre stage. "A contribution need not be understood; it need only be repeated, reproduced, forwarded. Circulation is the context, the condition for the acceptance or rejection of a contribution" (59). This generalised shift away from content (sign) towards circulation (signal) is today a central condition of both speech and action that we must reckon with.

But for the sake of introduction, allow me to bracket machinic fluency and focus on the more common, therapeutic, sense. The medical-industrial complex has thoroughly naturalised this register of fluency such that communication disabilities represent a diminished form of being. We could here consider a vast range of "voices": from the nonspeaking voices of people who are cognitively disabled or autistic, to the dysfluent speech of stutterers and those with cleft palate, the vocal tics induced by Tourette's, the "slurring tongue" of cerebral palsy (Clare 2017, 6), or aphasic speech. There are important differences (of access needs and access to support) across these examples. But what is common to disabled speech, in its many expressions, is an assumed unintelligibility that results in an unevenly distributed failure to be recognised as a rational and human (political) agent. Disabled speech with its dyslexic syntax and its temporal breaks, juts, or repetitions is disorienting and confusing within spheres of communication presumed to be frictionless. Against the technocratic view that renders dysfluency an object of medical-scientific rather than political knowledge, I read dysfluency as a form of biological plurality made into a biopolitical problem by imperatives of fluency.

Unlike the stutterer whose face convulses in an attempt to wrestle phonemes into the common world, we assume the fluent (that is normal, unmarked) speaker to exercise sovereign control over their body. The notion that fluency is characterised by effortless speech reflects, I suggest, what Hasana Sharp (2011, 44) refers to as the "artisanal" or "craftsman" model of speech wherein the body's actions are the mere externalisation of either "preformed reason or transparent intention." This is a deeply humanist idea, one where speech is the direct manifestation of individual agency. For Maurizio Lazzarato (2014, 68), the production of "distinct and individuated speakers" and linguistic interaction are both modelled on economic exchange and the juridical contract: rational agents entering into a contractual agreement. Technologies of fluency facilitate the fluid transaction between necessarily predefined and stable subjects who each speak and act with a univocal, rational voice. In this way, liberal humanism conceives the voice as a reflection of the humanist self, a "mirror of the soul" (Mazzei and Jackson 2017, 1091) that must be biopolitically legible.

Sharp's project and mine intersect. In *Spinoza and the Politics of Renaturalization*, she argues for a nonhumanist politic carefully attuned to the multiple forces that enable and constrain "preformed reason or transparent intention" (44). It comes as no surprise (at least for someone who speaks dysfluently) that Sharp begins her project of re-naturalisation with the tongue—the dragon guarding the humanist door:

> The craftsman model governs our views of speaking as much as our notions of making (transforming matter in accordance with the demands of spirit). We believe that we deliberate internally and proceed to externalize our mental process in the form of speech. Speech is treated as an expression, a publication of our interiority. On this artisanal model, ideas precede and govern actions, thoughts precede utterances, and minds command tongues. (43)

The artisanal model hides the *becoming* of speech such that the voice simply appears in the world as a certainty; this model thereby occludes those material, contingent, and local powers of any communicative milieu that both enable and constrain action. The artisanal model renders speech an instrumental function that conveys preformed meanings efficiently. This is a thoroughly sterile ecology of communication: minds making speech to transfer information to other minds.

More strongly: the liberal-humanist voice is constituted through a form of alienation, an abstraction from the social relations, affordances, collective voices, and environments that constitute the individual voice. The alienation of our voices has a history. We pretend that communication (if it must have a body) has a normal body: an abled body that needs no help, thank you very much; a male and virile body that dominates weakness and uncertainty to command attention; a straight body never veering from its course; a respectable white body that can be trusted to deliver civilised truths. When we're feeling our best, communication sheds the body altogether to become a direct link between minds, a psychic postal man. John Durham Peters (1999, 16) describes the widespread buzz about communication in the nineteenth century as the desire for "telepathy," the unmediated contact between and communion of souls. Telepathy is a dream invented circa 1880 by white bourgeois men afraid of the sin of voices playing together in the dirt.

The object of fear is the cripple: a word, Jay Dolmage (2013, 103) writes, "related to the Old English *creopan*, or *creep*, a word with slowness built into its vowels, but also a word that locates bodies, literally, in the dirt—moving with the belly on the ground" (emphasis in original). The history of speech-language pathology represents a process of purifying the voice and rendering it accelerable, compliant to market temporalities. The history of information and communication technologies represents a process of erecting information highways above the shit. In short, the craftsman model interprets speech not as a relational-collective *action* but as a technical—and ultimately technocratic—*making* (what Arendt calls a *poesis*) divorced from its material sites of enunciation. Emptied of its becoming, communication becomes highly optimisable, a matter of control from beginning to end.

From this vantage, allow me to return to the "problem" I introduced above of the dysfluent repetition. It is hard to overstate that being caught in deadly repetitions (like the inability to leave one's house due to shame) is a live worry for the disability community, especially when living under neoliberalism. Being denied access to flows of material, social, and discursive support is, to borrow Lauren Berlant's (2007, 761) phrase, a process of "slow death" where "populations [are] marked out for wearing out." But part of the issue is how we understand the concepts of repetition and danger, and whether we foreground these concepts against a larger ecological crisis. Thinking with Deleuze and Guattari, I suggest that our anxieties about vortices are often misdirected. Perhaps it is not dysfluency but fluency that ensnares life with a type of deathly repetition. For his own part, Deleuze (1990, 153) was particularly concerned with the homogenising tendencies of information and communication technologies to churn out repetition without difference: talking heads that ask the same questions and reproduce the same ideas, the same desires, the same forms of life. Guattari (2000) worried in a complementary way that capitalism transforms the world in its image both extensively—e.g., colonising space, and intensively—e.g., infiltrating the subconscious. In this double movement capitalism erodes at once environmental, social, and mental ecologies. Any emancipatory struggle must thus be staged for Guattari at the transverse of these three ecologies, and it follows that an irreducibly existential struggle resides at the heart of any critical praxis, one that, he argues, movements sometimes ignore at their peril. Capitalism, he writes:

> [d]emands that all singularity must be either evaded or crushed in specialist apparatuses and frames of reference. Therefore, it endeavors to manage the worlds of childhood, love, art, as well as everything associated with madness, pain death, or a feeling of being lost in the Cosmos. . . . Capitalistic subjectivity seeks to gain power by controlling and neutralizing the maximum number of existential refrains. (50)

Medical and therapeutic apparatuses neutralise the singularity of the voice—flattening its *this*ness and multiplicity (its redundancies, fissures, and connections) into humdrum binaries of normal/abnormal that can be represented and managed without remainder. Within this sterilised ecology, talking heads and trolls flourish but precarious forms of life get crushed in binaries such as self-hatred or self-acceptance.

Guattari's simplest example of a refrain is the songbird that creates a territory—a space of existence and belonging—through a chirping, singular repetition. It is noteworthy that the use of neonicotinoid insecticides and general ecological collapse has decimated the North American songbird population since the '70s, effectively silencing a vast choir of refrains (Pindar and Sutton 2000, 7). Across the same period, measures of neoliberal austerity have rendered the material worlds of disability communities increasingly bare, uninhabitable, austere (Goodley 2014; McRuer 2018). Taking these uninhabitable environments as evidence of pathological maladaptation, so-called specialists and armchair specialists pollute *social* and *mental* ecologies with endless repetitions of disableist and eugenic drivel, eroding the cultural imagination until an existence of disabled life outside of normative frameworks is hardly thinkable, yet alone liveable! Here, pollution manifests in noise rather than in silence, but it can result in a similar existential contraction where people can lack support of numerous kinds to generate or experiment with refrains. It is thus not only inefficiencies of the voice but vectors of subjectivity that are at stake in the discussion of fluency—the sites where new modes of subjectivity, intersubjectivity, and kinship might be cultivated. It is possible for dysfluency to mobilise a line of flight, though wobbly and uncertain.

To maintain at least the *fiction* of transparent flow depends on the continual upkeep of communication channels: dredging biopolitical debris and streamlining the environment. Robert McRuer and Anna Mollow (2012, 30) argue that "[n]eoliberal capital is fascinated *in general* with the ways that subgroups might be made more profitable and less dangerous or disruptive" (emphasis in original). Eugenics itself has always been a project of streamlining life, and accordingly traffics in problems of fluid dynamics such as turbulence and flow. It both annihilates unpredictable (and thus coded dangerous) vortices of life and guides them back into productive flows. Perhaps, then, the fear of the dysfluent eddy that circulates time and meaning out of place is more a fear of what Guattari (2000, 45) calls "counter-repetition": a vector of subjectivisation that "runs counter to the 'normal' order of things . . . an intensive given which invokes other intensities to form new existential configurations." A counterrepetition reworks an event to introduce a difference within repetition and release the virtual potentials of an assemblage. There are political and existential questions at stake that are difficult even to articulate within a surge of cheap talk: What might a dysfluent event become if not immediately managed within technocratic channels of communication? How might we relate differently? What might we become? Dysfluency is interesting not as a case study of breakdown but as a disclosure of the asymmetries of power and the declensions of freedom that structure our collective environments of speech.

There is one final question proper to address in the introduction: Why focus on neoliberalism? The production of fluent speech, let alone its function as passcode into the polis, is a phenomenon that stretches across the history of Western philosophy. Why not Aristotle, who posits an ideal human form? Why not Locke or Dewey, who long for perfect communication? Why not

Hobbes, so fearful of the multiple voice? That there are many starting points for a project to dethrone the head speaks to the head's instability. Nevertheless, I focus on neoliberalism for two primary reasons. First, neoliberalism arguably *is* the power to govern life via the excitation and control of mass assemblages of communicative bodies, and while the nomenclature around the current iteration of capitalism varies, for the sake of simplicity, I will refer to it as "info-capitalism."[1] Neoliberalism is what I call an "info-therapeutic" regime, the very machinery of cheap talk. Related, and second, I hope to contribute a "history of the present" (Foucault 1995, 31) that might help us attend to the political-existential-ecological urgency of our current moment.

Outline

This book is the product of an odd phenomenology, a description of the givenness of cheap talk within domains of life both organic and machinic. It begins with the familiar (the experience of cheap talk at work) and navigates through more alien yet ever-present manifestations of those "forces making us say things when we've nothing much to say" (Deleuze 1990, 137). The book is thus also a rough cartography, an attempt to map the relations of force and power that constitute cheap talk. The first three chapters examine, in turn, three biopolitical apparatuses that govern the communicative body. The first chapter concerns the therapeutic regime of speech-language pathology, the second the communication and information sciences of cybernetics, and the third chapter their collision—what I call "info-therapeusis." The final chapter offers tentative suggestions to broaden the range of political action beyond the framework of cheap talk.

In the first chapter, I argue that capitalism has put speech to work and made it a low-cost (i.e., cheap) stream of labour and human capital. Informational capitalism needs fluent info-workers, whom Clare Butler (2014) calls "straight talkers," and yet the biopolitical mechanisms by which humans have been disciplined to fit within the rhythms of informational capitalism have either been assumed and/or overcoded with ableist assumptions. This chapter, as such, traces the production of the fluent subject in the late-nineteenth and early-twentieth century and suggests that an articulate and fluent population emerges through the discourse and industry of speech-language pathology that seeks to make the capacity of speech manageable, efficient, and productive. In conclusion, I examine how neoliberalism captures fluency as a mode of human capital.

The second chapter turns from the domain of the human subject and labour to examine the distinctly machinic transformations that information societies (what Deleuze [1992] terms "societies of control") enact on the social field and communication itself. Control societies dissolve bodies into informational terms that get managed by filtering unwanted noise from the system. In this way, cybernetics depoliticises communication and seeks to render disability an inert force. And yet, I suggest with New Materialists Jane Bennett and Hasana Sharp that the tongue is ultimately uncontrollable—not governed by the will but activated by proximate bodies in our world. The "problem" of dysfluency is thus not really one of communication but of tenuous control over unruly bodies.

The third chapter mobilises the theory of the first two chapters to interrogate the talking head. The talking head is the product of info-therapeutics, of individualising therapeutic technologies in conjunction with the de-individualising informatic technologies of "machinic enslavement"—a term borrowed from cybernetics that refers to the management of component parts (Deleuze and Guattari 1987, 458). Info-therapeutics tunes speech-language pathology to the parameters of communication machines—this is what I call "machinic fluency." I moreover suggest in this chapter that the *function* of talking heads is to constitute a "universal priesthood" of communication that papers over declensions of neoliberal power. In conclusion, I take up Deleuze and Guattari's (1987, 500) warning to "[n]ever believe that a smooth space will suffice to save us" in the context of access to information and universal design.

In the final chapter I revisit the talking head, troll, and dysfluent speaker in consideration of the "crisis of truth-telling" produced by cheap talk, or what Foucault (2001) would call the crisis of parrhesia. In the ancient Greco world, parrhesia—honest, open, or courageous speech—was the civil duty of the Athenian aristocracy: speaking the truth for the good of the populace. However, the rise of democracy flooded the assembly with citizens and political voices. When everyone has access to the stage, could the voices of the truth-tellers be recognised? My conclusion thus seeks a positive critique of cheap talk: to expand the range of what *counts* as political action for dysfluent voices and to seek resources that can generate critical breaks within neoliberal modes of power. I accordingly map four possible modes of truth-telling within the lexicon of parrhesia: therapeutic (authentic), Platonic (rational), mischievous (trolling), and Cynic (shitting in the street). Taking up the motto of the Cynics—"deface the currency"—perhaps dysfluent voices can find resources to "de-face" speech and its mythic power, which has become entwined with capital. In this way, dysfluency might be a parrhesiastic *resource* rather than an impediment. By rethinking agency and truth-telling in terms of noncommunication rather than intelligibility, the unspeakable rather than the easily-said, disabled voices can expand the range of political action—and perhaps reclaim it from troll and talking head alike.

One

Putting Fluency to Work

Disabled subjects fail to embody the impossible norms of productivity that constitute industrial and postindustrial labour. It is true that even the ostensibly "able-bodied" fail to meet these norms, yet in neoliberal societies the presence of disability is prefigured as a failure of value, citizenship, and human identity. But what if we flipped the script? What if the disabled body is not a lack but a site of unruly agency? What if sluggish tongues don't *fail* at compulsory able-bodiedness but rather *refuse* its terms? I structure this chapter around the logic of refusal: the refusal of bodies to submit to capitalist systems of infinite production, the body's refusal to be made intelligible and articulate, the tongue's refusal to be governed.

Vignette 3: Bartleby, the Scrivener.

Herman Melville's ([1853] 1995) "Bartleby, the Scrivener: A Story of Wall Street" is the tale of a curious scribe who gets a job with a lawyer. Bartleby seems to be the ideal info-worker: meticulous, efficient, not distractible. But only during the morning. After lunch he becomes energetic, spilling ink and making noise. The lawyer tolerates this afternoon behaviour because of Bartleby's otherwise extraordinary labouring value. Yet one day, Bartleby begins an odd form of passive resistance, responding to each request with the simple phrase: "I would prefer not to." Any attempt to motivate Bartleby, or, as the story progresses and the anxiety of the employer increases, to remove him from the office, is met with the impassive wall: "I would prefer not to." From where does this stubborn refusal arise? Is he somehow disabled? Would it matter?

Vignette 4: Straight Talkers.

In "Wanted—Straight Talkers: Stammering and Aesthetic Labour," Clare Butler (2014), a sociologist of work, reports the lived experiences of thirty-six males[1] who stutter in work environments that are increasingly communicative. Says Brian, one participant: "I mean there's loads of things I can do, why don't they think about that. There's more to work than talking straight isn't there? Some straight talkers talk rubbish but that's alright is it?" (724). Although straight speech may in fact be a conduit for bullshit, to speak dysfluently is nevertheless a disqualifying mark within work contexts that require talk. Butler notes that "their level of fluency directly impacted on whether their message was heard and acted upon" (725) by coworkers and customers alike. Dysfluency disqualifies one as a speaker *not* because a person who stutters cannot transmit information, but because they cannot do so in a certain, fluent way that sets people at ease and deftly navigates complex social codes.

Simon, a different participant, notes how the dysfluent voice exposes the boundaries of social groups: "What's an interview for other than to find out if you'll fit in? Yes, it's about being able to do the job but it's more than that, it's will you fit with us, do I like you, will the team like you, and the clients, customers will they actually listen to you, respect you" (723). His speech is disqualified from work because it fails to embody normative codes of communication and styles of affective labour that delineate the boundaries of social groups. Recognising that hireability and promotion depend more and more on "talking straight," many of her participants felt burdened by the emotional labour of performing fluency in the workplace. "However," Butler continues, "they typically considered that this effort toward speech fluency is necessary and that this quest for sounding right is right, despite its frustrations" (728). The embodied work—the strenuous effort—of transforming one's speech (one's self) to meet able-bodied norms of verbal communication is taken to be an unfortunate yet necessary project.

• • •

The earnest claim that "[t]here's more to work than talking straight" seems less true all the time. Like many people with "a speech impediment," I spent, as part of my therapeutic training, many adolescent hours in a cramped room with only a speech-language pathologist (SLP) and a telephone—meeting my weekly quota of pathologising fake calls to local businesses. I would stutter made-up requests to unknown combatants over the line, suffering shame and embarrassment to "work on my fluency." How I hated that room. (People who stutter often feel a strong loathing for technologies such as the phone where communication relies almost entirely on the voice.) I experienced dread each week thinking about the SLP whose disciplinary presence and notepad would—not unlike the automatic dialing of call-centre systems—force me to keep dialing even when during the last conversation I had wavered near tears. Although I had not yet connected the dots, this discipline of my speaking body was of course job training for a postindustrial economy as investment in my communicative capital. The desirability of fluency on the telephone was never in question. Butler writes that unlike many other disabilities, stuttering is not accommodated at work. People expect accommodations for various forms of communication difference (Braille, screen readers, etc.), but not for disqualifying performances of speech. Perhaps fluent speech is today simply too essential for work. Maybe the postindustrial workplace cannot do without straight talkers.

My own experience reflects Kevin Paterson's (2012, 172) cautious suggestion that "the remit of speech and language therapy is to increase the physical and cultural capital of people with speech impairments." Speech therapy meant to wrestle my body into submission. Everyone hoped I was to become a good info-worker, a straight (and happy?) talker. But somewhere along the way, the work of trying to perform compulsory fluency became too much. While it is true that, at least in some environments, nearly any stutterer can achieve fll-lueeenccyyyy iiiiiiiiiffffffff tttttttthhhhhheeeeyyyyy slllooooooooooowwww doooooowwwwwnn tooooooooo siiiiiiiiiixxxxxxxttttyyyy ssssyyyyyyylllll-labbbbbblllleess ppeeeeeererrrr miiiiiinnnnutttttte, a person ends up sounding robotic and thus still not truly human. As I discuss in the next chapter, I tried a SpeechEasy—an in-ear delayed auditory feedback device that tricks the brain into fluency—but the world sounded like noise. And I simply did not care to self-discipline my body each day with therapeutic techniques in order to strive for normalcy. Fluency was something I never attained; my tongue simply preferred not to be capitalised.

Perhaps Bartleby and people who stutter have much in common. Despite his machinelike repetition, Bartleby is perhaps the farthest from a "straight talker" one can imagine. His hyper capacities are unreliable: irreducible to a stable and manageable stream of work. His embodied presence resists capitalisation. For Deleuze (1997, 73), "[Bartleby's] formula stymies all speech acts, and at the same time, it makes Bartleby a pure outsider to whom no social position can be attributed." There is something terribly odd about his character, for despite attempts to manage Bartleby as a labouring subject, his motives and identity remain utterly inscrutable. This existential impenetrability and intractability sends off warning bells within the halls of liberal capitalism. Turning resistant (dysfluent, disabled, and otherwise unruly) bodies into labour power is a difficult-enough task for the bourgeoise; "I would prefer not to" is a managerial nightmare.

We can track this embodied refusal to work at a macro register. Theorists in the Italian Autonomous (neo-Marxist) tradition insist that the creative impulse behind the automation of factories and the surge in information and communication technologies (ICTs) during the mid-twentieth century lies not with capital but with workers. Italian Autonomism is accordingly a "*workerist*" (or "*operaist*" in Italian) praxis insofar as it highlights the embodied powers of labour. The revolution of the production process, the Autonomists argue, is a *reaction* to the living and subjective power of labour. Theorists and activists such as Mario Tronti, Antonio Negri, and Paolo Virno accordingly locate the beginnings of post-Fordism in the joint student-worker strikes and sabotages in France and Italy in the '60s and '70s. The Bartlebian refusal to work (to show up or to work with any efficiency/compliance) as a site and strategy of resistance is where the term "workerism" comes from. It is this active yet passive refusal, they argue, that has forced capital's hand to develop and integrate automated machines and information and communication technologies into the mode of production. Always a mixed blessing, innovations such as automated assembly lines replace human labour as the main force of production, which in turn requires human attendants with "intellectual" capacities to oversee and regulate the process. This movement frees living labour to engage in more conversational, social, and ostensibly "human" work in the tertiary and quaternary sectors.

Drawing a line between these three narratives—Bartleby, "straight talkers," and the "productivist" agency of the Italian workerist tradition—helps frame the goals of this chapter.

The most immediate goal is to highlight the therapeutic regime of SLP and its biopolitical function to organise and insert tongues, brains, and voices into both capitalist machinery and social life. All three of these narratives represent resistance to biopolitical control that therapeutics might shore up.

The secondary goal is to reflect on the agency such refusals might afford. To imagine Bartleby as a workerist saboteur is to highlight the tension between productivism and antiproductivism within this form of agency, and really *any* refusal to work. It is a basic contradiction of capitalism that, in Dan Goodley's (2014, 169) words, it "produce[s] in excess of [its] practices." Put otherwise, "Neoliberalism and neoliberal-ableism cannot stop themselves from producing versions of dis/ability and humanness that can be seized upon by global citizens for their own ends, dependent of course upon their socio-economic position and their access to material, economic, cultural and social capital" (2014, 169). Neoliberalism needs straight speech and lots of it. But producing more possibility for contact always brings the possibility for subversion and unlikely alliances in unlikely ways—these are the excesses of neoliberalism that can be "worked" (33) towards radical ends. Let me be clear: disabled people are disproportionately exploited and dispossessed around the world. As Sunaura Taylor (2004) explains, "For many disabled people employment is unattainable. We often simply make inefficient workers, and inefficient is the antithesis of what a good worker should be. For this reason, we are discriminated against by employers." Access to employment and employment rights for disabled people remain necessary struggles. But, as Taylor herself insists when she argues for a "right not to work," there is simultaneously nonproductivist agency to be found in the excess of neoliberal ableism (agency that neoliberalism struggles to grasp) that we would be remiss not to consider.

Crip spaces and temporalities that emerge from the refusal of normativity can facilitate new modes of connection. This is political work, for as Robert McRuer (2012) writes, "We are continually generating a multitude of ways of being queer and crip, and of coming together. If we hope for another world that is not possible but livable, we can and should continue to generate more." Keeping in mind this crip desire for new modes of contact and being, we might ask: What are the differences, really, between Bartleby's refusal and the dysfluent resistance and/or refusal to communicate?[2] How different are the systems of discipline that try to contort both Bartleby and dysfluent speakers into straight lines? And what "yes" might the Bartlebian refusal enable? There are important alliances that still need to be made within the "undercommons" (Moten and Harney 2013) by the refuse of neoliberal capitalism.

This chapter maps the material and discursive conditions that gave rise to the straight talker. To do so, it follows the movement from industrial to postindustrial capitalism and denaturalises the organisation and insertion of tongues, brains, and voices into capitalist machinery. The faculties and subject of communication did not simply show up for work one day fully formed; "communicative competency" as a generic ability—a distinct and ableist mode of human capital—has a history that must be grasped before resistance to the lure of info-capitalism can be thought.

Fluency at Work

Industrial-age manufacturing, or so-called "Fordism," flourished in America during the late nineteenth century and constructed, Michael Hardt (1999,

93) explains, a "relatively 'mute' relationship between production and consumption" where "[t]he mass production of standardized commodities in the Fordist era could count on an adequate demand and thus had little need to 'listen' closely to the market." Fordist labour can likewise be understood as a relatively "mute" activity. Epitomised by work in factories before relentless assembly lines, industrial labour creates value through the repetition of standardised and calculable motions. It is the systematic expenditure of bioenergy representable in the abstract form of labour-power.

Industrial labour makes human conversation *difficult* because factory machines are loud, and *redundant* insofar as the factory rationalises the process of work to make talk and social interaction as unnecessary as possible. Paolo Virno (2001) writes that, compared to cottage industries, industrial "[p]roduction is a silent chain, where only a mechanical and exterior relation between what precedes it and what follows it is allowed, whilst any interactive correlation between what is simultaneous to it is expunged." In early factory systems, the level of cooperation and communication needed to carry out tasks was simple enough that the panoptical gaze of the foreman in the centre of the factory floor could bind silent workers to their quotas. Intersubjective communication was displaced in and thus contained by this gaze and the route systems of tasks assigned to individual workers by the foreman. Excluding the capacity to relay basic orders or warn of danger, communicative ability was more or less extraneous to the process of valorisation for workers on the factory floor.

In contrast to Fordism and its logic of massification and standardisation, the model of post-Fordism is often called "just-in-time" production and aims to produce only as much stock as is currently needed. From manufacturing, to telecommunications, to public relations, to neoliberal education factories, to financial industries, the agile production and consumption of *information* has become essential to survive in hypercompetitive global markets. The labouring practices of post-Fordist industries are similarly characterised by the flexible capacity to produce and consume information. Here we might think of social media influencers, or gig labourers such as Uber drivers, contract teachers, and freelance copywriters. It is important to note that the shift that Butler and others track towards aesthetic and communicative labour is part of the ubiquitous informatisation of social life. "The inclusion of 'essential: excellent communication skills' as a requirement in the person specification of a job application pack would result in little shock and invoke minimal outrage" (Butler 2014, 719–20). Much to the dismay of dysfluent speakers, communication is increasingly expected rather than shunned at work, such that post-workerists such as Paolo Virno and Lazzarato argue that post-Fordism should be defined as the transition from "mute" to "chatty" labour—the inclusion of sociality within productive networks.

With Butler, but extending her analysis, I suggest in this chapter that we focus on the mode and production of the ideal info-labourer via therapeutic techniques. The labouring subject no longer produces value simply as a reliable source of energy, but as a stable nexus of information: the post-Fordist worker (such as the Uber driver) is a distinctly communicative and affective entity who must be capable of connecting, channeling, and redirecting productive flows—while always increasing its brand. The circulation of info-capital demands that workers become proper "subjects of communication" (Lazzarato 1996, 135) whether or not they are producing immaterial commodities. As communicative processes are increasingly incorporated in all labour practices, the *need* for straight talkers who can adapt flexibly to multiple temporalities grows—as does the stigma when body-minds refuse to submit.

It is here important to recognise with Jason Read (2003, 84) that abstract labour is not a passive and homogenised capacity, but a docile mode of the active and unruly force possessed by human subjects to create something new, an excessive power that the bourgeoisie must continually reduce and discipline into a calculable energy. Marx (1976, 290–91) refers to this generative capacity as "living labour." As Read (2003, 17) argues, capitalism must produce *while constraining* the abstract capacity to work, developing the "potentiality of the subjectivity of labour while at the same time reducing the possibility for conflict and antagonism." With the exponential growth of industrial manufacturing in the early twentieth century, factory owners mobilised the technology of Taylorisation, or "scientific management," to mechanise and de-skill the labouring process and thereby minimise the collective capacity for resistance while also optimising the interface between workers and machines. Yet what is the factory but a site of ever-possible disorderliness, a system prone to spring leaks of both energy and desire? A primary aspect of living labour is creativity, sociality, cooperation, and communicability. The mechanisation of labour simply leaves the worker with more time to think (nonconformist thoughts). And as workers were gathered in factories, they formed increasingly complex networks of cooperation, constituting yet exceeding the mode of production that capitalism must continually displace and suppress.

The body must be disciplined to both produce and consume precisely because "[t]he body is *the place* through which capital moves" (Goodley 2014,

91; emphasis in original). But as we have already seen, the body also resists this process of capitalisation—the grinding of living into abstract labour—and it is here that disabled body-minds represent a spectral limit to capital accumulation. Disability represents the entropy or heat death of infinite production that capitalism has sought to stave off with technologies of segregation, co-option, or now, therapeusis. The unyielding rhythm of industrial machines bound to the logic of capitalist valorisation standardised the body in relation to the norm of the "average worker" (Davis 1996, 28–29) and thereby spawned a multitude of deviant subjects. Industrial workers were exploited for their thermodynamic energy indexed against rigid bio-industrial norms that excluded from participation many people who were identified as blind, deaf, chronically ill, and otherwise physically or intellectually disabled. "The new [industrialized] process of production demanded a form of somatic flexibility," writes Kevin Paterson (167), "that was determined by the pace and rhythm of the mechanized factory floor rather than the individual worker." Thus the energy of bodies that could not, for example, stand for long periods of time and make repetitive motions could not easily be consolidated and put to use in most factory systems.

Maintaining a highly exploitable workforce demands a categorisation of biologically legitimated difference that can be used administratively to segregate charity from productive subjects. "By focusing on curing so-called abnormalities, and segregating those who could not be cured into the administrative category of 'disabled,'" Marta Russell and Ravi Malhotra (2002, 214) explain, "medicine cooperated in shoving less exploitable workers out of the mainstream workforce. So, just as capitalism forces workers into the wage relationship, it equally forcefully coerces disabled workers out of it." Capitalism has always found use for its losers. Since the energy of disabled bodies was not easily exploitable, an ontology of abnormalcy cast their bodies outside the factory walls as objects of pity and need. But, as Brendon Gleeson (1999, 108) writes, by the late nineteenth century, many people assumed to be unfit for work had been incarcerated in "a new institutional system of workhouses, hospitals, asylums, and (later) 'crippleages.'" Disability is in this way a social and political category used to sort human difference according to the needs of capitalist production, a category that emerges as a social problem (to be managed by a state and para-state apparatus) set against the ceaseless demands of industrial capitalism.

As I explore further in the next chapter, neoliberalism produces losers with more granularity by dissolving rigid binaries such as normal/abnormal into processes of differential inclusion. That "[t]here is no such thing as an 'adequately abled' body anymore" (Puar 2013, 182) means, Anne McGuire and Kelly Fritsch (2019, 92) explain, that "the key question of the normal body in the 21st century is not 'Is this a normal body or not?' but rather '*How* normal is this body; how amenable is it to normative enhancements or optimization?'" This new normal, they continue, is more inclusive than its industrialised predecessor since it can flexibly include in its count "abnormal" or "non-average" bodies such as racialised, disabled, and queer bodies, but *if and only if* such bodies and minds "can be captured by market rationality, or market values" (Fritsch 2015, 29). In other words, one must be the right kind of disabled subject to find inclusion within neoliberal societies—productive or profitable in some other way. It is such that postindustrial labour opens some new possibilities for disabled labour while also producing disability through exploitative relations that enhance some at the expense of others.

Nevertheless, as Jon Beasley-Murray (2010) writes of attempts to maintain hegemonic control, "something always escapes!" This implies, in one regard, a subversive possibility for disabled bodies precisely because they are more difficult to exploit. Sunaura Taylor (2004) explains that since disabled people have been kept from work and thus neoliberal value, "[d]isabled people have to find meaning in other aspects of their lives and this meaning is threatening to our culture's value system."

In a similar regard, "something always escapes!" means that living labour refuses to be silenced. "As the number of co-operating workers increases," explains Marx (1976, 449), "so too does their resistance to the domination of capital, and, necessarily, the pressure put on by capital to overcome this resistance." Increasingly complex production generates collective power that resists capital: this is a basic contradiction of capitalism. Industrialisation falters in its attempt to achieve total control over the intellectual, creative, social, and communicative power of the human subject. The capitalist mode of production characterised as Taylorism and Fordism mobilises communication while remaining external to it—what is termed "a formal subsumption of communication." A real subsumption, or an internal restructuring of social relations to bring communication within the capitalist mode of production, was needed to grasp living labour more fully. In other words, capitalism needed to produce subjectivities of communication.

Cognitive Capitalism and the Virtuoso

The term "cognitive capitalism" is adopted by post-workerists such as Paolo Virno and Christian Marazzi. This is a specific reading of info-capitalism, one that focuses *signifying* semiologies operative at the *subjective* level. Cognitive capitalism routes the heterogeneous set of productive activities that make up so-called "immaterial labour" through the human subject and through language. This tenet is simultaneously its greatest strength and weakness. In their favour, Virno and Marazzi diversify the discussion in post-workerism beyond technical machinery to show that socialised knowledge has also taken root in the bodies and social interactions of workers themselves. Virno (2004, 60), for example, argues that labour is increasingly defined by the "spectacle" of communication. Cognitive capitalism puts language to work twice insofar as linguistic action is both the product *and* the means of labouring activity. The media, health, education, service, and various other sectors of the economy attest to the duality of communication at work; the "raw materials" of language are deployed in social interactions and are immanently transformed through their use into a spectacle as semiotic products (Marazzi 2008, 50). Yet I nevertheless suggest that cognitive capitalism naturalises communicative capacity—what Virno refers to as the pure "ability to speak"—insofar as it posits a quasi-formal rather than real subsumption of communicative subjectivity.

In his articulation of communicative labour, Virno (2004) mobilises the concept of "virtuosity," which denotes excellence within the performing arts. The meaning or purpose of a virtuosic activity is always immanent to its performance such that virtuosity requires, by necessity, the presence of others for its fulfillment.[3] Like singing or acting, the performance of human language has its fulfillment in itself: it does not produce an external object and requires the presence of others in a publicly organised space. For Virno, what sets the speaker apart from other virtuosos is that she, making use of the *potentiality* of language, requires no script (56). A singular utterance is determinate—manifesting a historical vernacular and grammar—but for Virno the *act* of speaking never follows a predetermined script. The so-called ability to speak and communicate exists as a pure *dynamis* or potentiality, guided only by the general intellect. The concept of "general intellect" is defined by Marx (1973, 626) as socialised knowledge that is objectified in fixed capital such as robotics. However, commentators like Virno recognise that general intellect is not merely congealed as technology but is also manifest in living labour. "We should consider the dimension," Virno writes (65), "where the general intellect, instead of being incarnated (or rather, cast in iron) into the systems of machines, exists as attributes of living labour. The general intellect manifests itself today, above all, as the communication, abstraction, self-reflection of living subjects." General intellect is externalised knowledge: thought made public as it is rendered productive.

It is worth recognising with Hardt the two faces of info-work: one "low-value" and the other high. Each implies its own formation of communicative capacity and process of subjectivisation. In the first mode, immaterial labour is constituted by the instrumentalised transmission of information, which in turn relies on normalised proficiency in reading, writing, hearing, and speaking. This is a deadened form of virtuosity in which "communicative action, human relations, and culture have been instrumentalised, reified, and 'degraded' to the level of economic interactions" (Hardt 1999, 96). Through mindless jobs like data entry, transcribing, delivering, and reproducing information at work, "the subject becomes a simple relayer of codification and decodification, whose transmitted messages must be 'clear and free of ambiguity'" (Lazzarato 1996, 134). These sorts of jobs can offer a type of holding space (and simultaneously, a haven) for dysfluent speakers in post-Fordist economies. Butler explains that as workplaces become more communicative, dysfluent speakers can get placed into lower-level, backroom positions (manual labour mixed with low-value info-labour) away from customers. The precariousness of the workplace for stutterers is itself valuable for employers, for as a fellow stutterer recently mourned, "Stutterers make good workers. We don't complain!"

Attending to such gradations within postindustrial labour disrupts the premise that twenty-first-century workplaces are straightforwardly more social and communicative. While the mute-to-chatty narrative is a useful starting point, it also tends to reify both idealised industrial workers (compliant and reliable sources of energy) and postindustrial workers (fluent nodes of information), and remove both from their smaller micropolitical and larger geopolitical contexts. It is here that neo-Marxists like George Caffentzis (2013) would point out that cognitive capitalism quite conveniently eclipses the grim network of sweatshops, chemical factories, and mining operations (not to mention click farms and call centres) in the Global South that make globalised information economies possible. Moreover, the premise of ever more communication in the workplace erases the productive role that a-sociality and a-communicability can play in info-capitalism. For example, Silicon Valley businesses have recently been hiring autistic folk to cash in on ableist narratives. "Two years ago, I didn't know anything about autism," says Hiren C. Shukla, a director of a multinational professional services network. "There is this rich, diverse pool of talent that is untapped" (Elias 2017). Working from the deeply harmful stereotypes that (a) autistics have social and communicative deficits that (b) they make up for with other skills, this hiring practice is framed as a good return on investment for labour as well as branding. Shukla concedes that their so-called autism training program also generates a "tremendous amount of reputational capital" (Elias 2017).

Keeping this mottled character of the "increasingly communicative" workplace in mind, Hardt (1999, 96) suggests that for the service industries, "communication has not been impoverished but rather production has been enriched to the complexity of human interaction." That is, in industries such as retail, health services, entertainment, or journalism, the true virtuoso does not simply transmit information but creates and modifies affect. Managers often shield dysfluent speakers from affective labour since this labour is "immaterial, even if it is corporeal and affective, in the sense that its products are intangible: a feeling of ease, well-being, satisfaction, excitement, passion—even a sense of connectedness or community" (Hardt 1999, 96). The virtuoso is decidedly fluent insofar as affective labour trades in aesthetically normalised human contact. The common fear, anxiety, and discomfort experienced in the presence of disability now lie thoroughly internal to the production of capital.[4]

Raising communicative labour to the level of human interaction thus demands far more of dysfluent subjects than instrumentalised communication. For a virtuosic labourer, it is not enough to transmit information: one must induce positive affect by communicating adeptly across the full range of human interactions. Hitting proper cues, tones, speeds, accents, body postures, facial expressions, and standing distances (not to mention writing styles and efficiency, grammar, and punctuation) are choreographies of communication (Paterson 2012; St. Pierre 2015) or microstrategies of the body mobilised to put interlocutors at ease and stimulate desire. "From an organizational viewpoint," writes Butler, "the function of aesthetic labour is to promote a positive image with the aim of achieving beneficial outcomes" (2014, 726). One cannot be a valuable affective worker if one fails to meet aesthetic norms that facilitate contact through normalised sociality.[5]

The normalising code of the virtuoso is also gendered. Butler cites research to explain that "man's talk"—the manner of speaking in the workplace that is coded as masculine—affirms hierarchical position, is dominant, directive, attention-seeking, controlling, assertive, clear, forceful, and direct (2014, 721). If gendered male, these characteristics must be performed successfully to have one's speech registered as full speech. The failure of straight-masculine speech (St. Pierre 2015) can perhaps lead to a becoming-minority. When Butler's "participants reported that they had developed these other attributes [heightened intuition and social awareness], they often referred to them as 'female traits' (Richard 40–49), 'more often seen in women, some might say' (Peter 30–39), or 'showing my feminine side' (Oliver 30–39)" (Butler 2014, 727). While other feminised norms of communication, such as "chattiness," that are useful in the post-Fordist workplace might not obtain, Butler's participants recognised value in stepping outside of masculinised social roles and modes of sensory comportment.

In short, it is not enough to claim with Virno (2004, 63) that "nobody is as poor as those who see their own relation to the presence of others, that is to say, their own communicative faculty, their own possession of a language, reduced to wage labor." Our productive relations to others do not reduce to operations of wage labour because they are also racialised, gendered, and shaped by ableism in ways that reproduce hegemonic and productive social structures.

The fluent and thoroughly naturalised voice might accordingly be understood as at worst complicit with, and at best a function of, the capitalist desire to individuate and make speech compatible with labour-power and surplus wage extraction as human capital. This taken-for-granted voice that communicates automatically and without friction is an uncoincidentally optimal medium for info-capital. The critical opening for a genealogy of fluent and productive speaking subjects comes through Virno's insistence that the "communication industry" or "culture industry" is the post-Fordist industry of the means of production:

> Traditionally the industry of the means of production is the industry that produces machinery and other instruments to be used in the most varied sectors of production. However, in a situation in which the means of production are not reducible to machines but consist of linguistic-cognitive competencies inseparable from living labour, it is legitimate to assume that a conspicuous part of the so-called "means of production" consists of techniques and communicative procedures. (2003, 61)

Virno identifies the industry of the means of production with the "culture industry" since the generic faculty is largely naturalised and removed from the equation. Thus, Virno's claim that the culture industry produces communicative procedures must be read *through* the production of fluent subjects, which is an industry that draws out and exploits ableist, classist, and neocolonialist norms and relations.

The Industry of the Means of Production: A Genealogy of Fluency[6]

My guiding question in this section is quite simple: How has speech been made into an object pliable to the operations of biopower and the interests of capital? How, more specifically, were fluent speaking subjects—straight talkers—produced? The production of biopolitical subjects never follows a straight and even path but emerges through the contestation of multiple and discordant forces (Foucault 1980). The stuttered movement towards a biopolitics of communication and postindustrial labour might accordingly be initially located in the tension between nineteenth-century education and elocutionary practices: between the desire for an articulate population and the desire to shore up class and race distinctions through "pure" speech.

Following the War of 1812, Americans increasingly turned towards "common" education as a manifestation of their civic virtues. Urbanisation and industrialisation, along with ostensible desires for class equality, contributed to the felt need for improved educational opportunities. In Foucauldian terms, "common" education coincides with the biopolitical need for well-rounded and governable subjects—and by extension, a population—rather than simply people occupying specialised occupations, such as doctors, lawyers, or ministers. Speech was concurrently emerging as a generic, as opposed to specialist, capacity central to American democratic and industrial society.[7] In step with the increasing centrality of the oral in this social milieu, American "educators began to popularize the needs of man as an articulate person in his practical world; they saw man as a citizen speaking as well as reading" (Borches and Wagner 1954, 285). Along with this information wave, a *dispositif*, or apparatus of power/knowledge, was needed to render the hitherto unruly capacity of speech manageable, efficient, and productive.

Constructing an articulate citizenry was difficult, however, and not simply due to the requisite social, discursive, and technical infrastructure. An articulate citizenry required norms against which speaking bodies could be measured and disciplined, and calculating these norms would be nearly impossible until compulsory education and child labour laws were passed in the early twentieth century (Simon 1954, 400); these, along with standardised tests and surveys, would enable vast amounts of data to be gathered on "normal" and "deviant" speech. Yet the antecedent issue is that defining and embodying norms of "proper" speech is a moving contradiction that at once seeks to contain *while* circulating differences in classed and racialised dictions, cadences, and grammars.

A central nineteenth-century site for cultivating legible speech in American educational institutions (and private practices) was elocution, a discipline that migrated from England, where it had earlier taken hold, in the mid-eighteenth century. One of its chief proponents in England, Thomas Sheridan (1762), had described the general state of verbal utterance with disdain:

> Amongst those who speak in the senate house, pulpit, or at the bar, as well as amongst men in private life, we find stammerers, lispers, a mumbling, indistinct utterance; ill management of the voice, by pitching it in too high or too low a key; speaking too loudly, or too softly as not to be heard; and using discordant tones, and false cadences. These being, I say, common to all ranks and classes of men, have not any marks of disgrace put upon them, but, on the contrary, meet with general indulgence from a general corruption. (32–33)

Motivated by anxieties of many stripes, elocutionists on both sides of the Atlantic took it upon themselves to improve the quality of spoken language. During the nineteenth century in the US, textbooks such as Ebenezer Porter's 1827 *Analysis of the Principles of Rhetorical Delivery as Applied in Reading and Speaking* and James Rush's *Philosophy of the Human Voice*, published in the same year, were widely used in public schools and private practices. Rush, the son of Dr. Benjamin Rush, arguably pioneered the science of the voice by applying his expertise in medicine to the speaking subject.[8] Others had described the anatomical structure of the speech mechanism, but Rush was the first to identify, through a systematic nomenclature, the physiology of speech production in relation to elements of the voice—force, pitch, quality, and rhythm (Hale 1949, 452). By rendering vocal expression an entirely describable and objective phenomenon, Rush enabled a science of vocal duration and succession to be mapped onto and habituated within the speaking body. Rush's methodological attention to the anatomy and physiology of the utterance was foundational for the future science of speech, but was often misread and dismissed in his time.

Speech education was thus taken up by departments of English and rhetoric in the second half of the nineteenth century, while elocution dropped to an elective status and migrated from public to private institutions (Nichols and Murphy 1954, 173). Despite this fact, and although they would be labelled the invention of "quacks" and "charlatans" (Van Riper 1939) by the forthcoming "scientific" speech correctionists, elocutionists offered some of the first curative programs for the speech defect that extend into the early twentieth century. Moreover, these curative techniques provide the basic anatomo-political structure for speech correction as it moves from a private practice to a social imperative.

It is crucial not to overlook the racial and class politics of these elocutionary practices. Elocutionists like Sheridan expressed a general concern about poor speech within the population as a whole, yet the predominant worry was illegible and uncultivated speech leaching into the habits and practices of the bourgeoisie. Dwight Conquergood (2000, 326) in this way reads elocution from the perspective of racial tension and class struggle. "Elocution expressed in another key the body-discipline so characteristic of industrial capitalism, but this was a discipline imposed on the bourgeoisie, a way for them to mark 'distinction' from the masses." The problem with the common word was precisely its commonality; elocution, Conquergood argues, was designed to recover the power of the spoken word from the masses—that is, to shore up the privilege of white property owners.

> Elocution sought to tap the power of popular speech but curb its unruly embodiments and refine its coarse and uncouth features. It was the verbal counterpart, on the domain of speech, of the enclosure acts that confiscated the open commons, so crucial to the hardscrabble livelihood and recreation of the poor, and privatized them for the privileged class. Elocution seized the spoken word, the common currency to which the illiterate poor had open access, and made it uncommon, fencing it off with studied rules, regulations, and refinements. (327)

The enclosure of the common word represents a type of tragedy of the commons. Subjection is always in step with hierarchy, and becoming a "refined" subject of language and speech reifies oneself as fully human (not animal), white (not Black), rich and educated (not poor and ignorant). A "proper" accent even today marks social class and connotes certain levels of intelligence, education, and respectability. Technologies of elocution habituated norms of "proper speech" within individual subjects who could then access social privilege and social mobility through the uncommon word.

The film *My Fair Lady*—originally George Bernard Shaw's *Pygmalion*—highlights how accent and speech pattern mobilise social power at the intersections of ability, gender, race, and class, both creating and marking communicative capital. In the film, Eliza Doolittle enlists the help of Professor Henry Higgins to transform her strong working-class accent into civilised and civilising English. Her desire is to work in a flower shop (labour that was precluded because of her improper speech); his is to prove that she can pass as civilized within elite English society. Kevin Paterson (2012, 173) writes of Higgins that "the traditional goal of speech and language therapy is to determine ways in which (carnal) performance of a person with speech impairment might be restored to something approximating the orderliness of 'proper communication.'" Proper speech alone does not grant social respectability or access to labour markets. But the carnal performance of speech casts a long shadow in the social imaginary. Especially in an increasingly digital age, the capacity of communicative competence—logocentrism refracted through numerous vectors of power—is perhaps the sine qua non of social power.

As Conquergood suggests above, elocution deploys a distinctly industrial capitalist set of biopolitical operations on the bourgeois body in this attempt to standardise and replicate vocal norms of class and civility. Yet while elocution was meant to enclose the commons, this enclosure leaked. Elocution was a technology that regulated and then recirculated the excess of orality, analogous to the work of the printer's type within scribal culture (326). Indeed, Conquergood cites Anna Russell's (1851, 15) *The Young Ladies' Elocutionary Reader*, where the uncultivated voice is described as an error, a smudge: "It resembles, in its effect to the ear, that presented to the eye, when the sheet has been accidentally disturbed in the press, and there comes forth, instead of the clear, dark, well-defined letter, executed distinctly on the fair white page, a blur of half-shade" (cited in Conquergood, 326).

One premise of this curious statement is that aberrations or "vocal smudges" exist only in relation to a system of standardisation and mechanisation. The attempt to standardise the speech patterns by which nineteenth-century subjects could access class privilege created and perpetuated the dilemma it sought to address. A slightly different way of stating this problem is that bourgeois speech, and the bourgeois speaking subject, is necessarily defined against the racial, classed, and disabled other. The excess of orality can never be eliminated, since it is an articulation of the necessarily public and political character of speech (Arendt 1998). Smudges on the voice are akin to grimy blurs on the face that bespeak a lower form of life, a life not fully human. An utterance will always be common or polyvocal; the bourgeois voice is thus not simply bordered by but shot through with the voices of the immigrant, the working class, and the dysfluent. As a result, creating a social factory of speech correction (albeit here in a nascent stage) that both cultivates and standardises the capacity of speech can only serve to circulate and proliferate the problem of excess and its correlate: the vocal deviant.

The vocal deviant is perhaps the key to understanding the post-Fordist industry of the means of production. Not only is "deviance" a constitutive aspect of the very capacity to speak, an excessive mode of the phonetic that cannot but trace the political edges of intelligibility and belonging, but for Foucault, the pathological has *methodological* primacy over the normal within any account of subjection. Despite its fall from grace as regime of truth, I suggest that elocution represents a font of modern strategies to render speech intelligible and manageable.[9] That is, consonant with the Foucauldian emphasis on the pathological over the normal, elocution was one of the first modern disciplines to problematise the "speech deviant" as a simultaneously social and individual problem, and by extension to objectify the voice and the speaking subject as a target of a scientific and medicalised *dispositif*.[10]

Speech Correction and Biopolitics

While elocution provides the initial momentum for the biopolitics of speech in America, its discursive and disciplinary hold on the speaking subject was held back by the embryonic state of the science and by a lack of social urgency. In a contestation for the truth of the speaking body, disciplines as heterogeneous as phonetics, medicine, education, psychology, psychoanalysis, and mental hygiene would absorb and transform the biopolitical impulse and anatomo-political technologies of elocution, setting them on an empirical and verifiable scientific footing. The result of this Foucauldian "game of truth" is the industry of speech-language pathology (SLP). Edward W. Scripture—a turn-of-the-century physician, phonetician, and experimental psychologist—embodies the fledgling science of speech that, significantly, cleaves along the lines of normalcy and abnormalcy:

> In most medical faculties no place is accorded to speech defects; the same is true in schools of pedagogy. This was formerly justified on the ground that a scientific study of speech and its defects did not exist. In the last decade, however, the science of phonetics has extended itself to laboratory work and university teaching; moreover, speech clinics have been established in several of the foremost medical schools. The treatment of these defects thus stands upon an entirely new basis; namely, that of a *carefully developed science of normal and pathological speech.* (1912, v; emphasis added)

Problematising speech in terms of normal/pathological enables the oral anxieties of class and race in the nineteenth century to be translated into a standard deviation and, through a series of knowledges and techniques, distributes speaking subjects hierarchically according to classifications. The "speech defective" thus becomes a reified subject, a target for biopolitical strategies of normalisation. Speech correction also constitutes the "normal speaker," who is necessarily caught in speech correction's hierarchical surveillance and normalising judgment. The faculty of speech is not only common but central to social and economic exchange. Resonant with the circulatory form of power that Foucault calls "security" (a point I take up more fully in the next chapter), the question for governing a capacity like speech is not so much "How can we isolate the speech defect?" as "How can we regulate the circulation of speech and cancel out its dangers?" (cf. Foucault 2007). Benjamin Bogue (1912), advertising his institute for stammerers, proclaims that "Our age demands perfect speech." This imperative necessarily implicates the entire population in a matrix of compulsory able-bodiedness. The abnormal, in other words, renders the biopolitics of speech intelligible yet was never its sole target. The management of speech and the production of fluid semiotic subjects must be located *through* the dysfluent, but within the entire social field.

Thus, it is important to note that while Scripture's (1912, 3) concern for the "speech defective" is largely one of charity—"The life of a stutterer," he writes, "is usually so full of sorrow that it can hardly be said to be worth living"—he also begins to problematise the speech defect in the biopolitical terms of economic cost and the good of society. Stutterers and lispers are imagined as an "irritating distraction to their teachers" and a "needless retardation to their classes" (v). One year earlier, in 1911, John Madison Fletcher (a stutterer, professor of psychology, and pioneer of SLP) states the threat of the speech defect for the education-factory even more starkly:

> If I understand the great movement for efficiency in commercial lines as Dr. Taylor and others have conceived it, the first point of attack is the sources of lost energies, misplaced efforts and neglected forces. In other words, the whole efficiency movement begins with the *stoppage of leaks, lost motions and costly frictions*. . . . If you should stand before a class in which there was a stuttering boy trying to recite, and watch this stumbling, halting, blushing and writhing embodiment of mental torture, and see the sympathy, worry, distraction of attention and anxiety of the teacher no less than the rest of the class, you could understand what I mean by this great leakage of energy. (148–49; emphasis added)

Invoking Taylorisation in the context of the speech defect is telling, to say the least, as it situates the speech defective within an industrialised system that regulates living labour. The "stoppage of leaks, lost motions, and costly frictions" refers in one regard to the smooth operation of the education-factory, yet it also refers to the production of semiotic subjects that are fluid, docile, and "interoperable" (Berardi 2009), or capable of interfacing with standardised semiotic systems. According to this productivist logic, the speech defect represents a costly friction—a leakage of useful energy and productive affect, an entropic force, the possibility of heat death—not just within the education-factory but across the social field.[11] Yet, as I explore in chapter 3, from the perspective of what Aimi Hamraie and Kelly Fritsch call "crip technoscience" (Hamraie 2017; Hamraie and Fritsch 2019), frictions can also constitute sites of generative possibility.

The concern over "leaked energy" and the regulation of speech as a biopolitical capacity foreshadows the internalisation of communication within capitalism and the emergence of speech as a form of human capital. The *problem* of the speech defect was not simply economic but one of life itself. Clarence Simon (1954, 406) suggests that speech correction lagged up until the twentieth century in part because educators had understood speech as a mere expression of the mind that did not aid its development. Psychology, however, established a relation between speech and ideation that flows both ways such that uncorrected speech could in fact *cause* deficient minds and personalities. The effect of this reversal, no matter its verity, was to place speech in the midst of the biopolitical struggle for life. Ira Wile (1916, 585), a physician, mental hygienist, and the commissioner of education in New York City, argues that speech defects "decrease the social worth of the individual and rob the community of the full fruits of human mentality." And speaking to the National Education Association (NEA) in 1916, James Green, the director of the New York Institute for Speech Defects, boldly claims: "Efficiency and ease seem to go together as a characteristic of mental strength and economy. 'Living at the tips of one's nerves' though an impediment of speech tends to develop vicious circles of nervous instability resulting in an increase of criminals, prostitutes, and general failures" (866). Psychology opened up the person to intervention by transforming the interiority of the soul into a set of "calculable traces" (Rose 2007, 74). The costly and leaky frictions of the speech-defective are thus not simply an economic loss, but a *danger* to society itself. Foucault's (1978, 7) claim that "nineteenth-century psychiatry was a medical science as much for the societal body as for the individual soul" obtains for the speech defect as well as the sexually abnormal.

In one regard, the problem of the speech defect is seemingly contained by the burgeoning scientific discipline of speech correction. In a state of biopolitical and eugenic fervour, Dr. Dennis J. McDonald (1916, 863), a commissioner of education in New York, spoke to the NEA and proclaimed that "Plans are under consideration whereby the board of education will provide in the very near future for its thousands of children suffering from defective speech, thus wiping out all handicaps and setting a standard for normal American children." Within these early years of speech correction, it was often assumed that speech defects could be outright eliminated, a eugenic hope buoyed by a scientific discourse that had ostensibly rendered speech a docile object primed for curative intervention. These "plans under consideration" include speech correction programs and speech clinics, which were cropping up across the country. Unsurprisingly, speech—a mode of living labour—was far more recalcitrant to disciplinary technologies than anticipated. By the 1930s, the discipline of speech correction increasingly shifted into a rehabilitative rather than curative mode that sought to make the speech defective socially useful since it could not be outright cured—bringing to mind Eli Clare's (2017, 10) quip that "Overcoming is cure's backup plan."[12] In addition, the number of US schoolchildren with "serious defects of speech" ballooned during this period, a result of more "accurate" technologies of calculation that continually narrowed the parameters of normal speech.

A primary reason speech correction is incapable of containing the speech defect, let alone eliminating it, is because—like elocution—speech correction circulates deviancy and produces the problem it seeks to solve. Yet this will ultimately be beneficial for the *dispositif* of speech correction, since it consolidates the discursive authority of speech correction across the social field. However striking McDonald's eliminativist desires may be, the second part of his claim, setting a standard for normal American children, is perhaps even more salient for the current discussion of the industry of means of production. The "correct" use of language establishes identitarian hierarchies, yet since "normal" speech is a biopolitical-statistical calculation that exists only within systems of equivalency, normalisation, and production, the normate (Garland-Thomson 1997) must be continuously reproduced through biopolitical technologies. Creating a standard for normal children in practice means generalising the biopolitical and, in turn, anatomo-political strategies used on those with speech defects across the population.

Targeting the "normal" population with speech-correction technologies follows Foucault's (1980, 102) insistence that "the bourgeoisie could not care less about delinquents, about their punishment and rehabilitation, which economically have little importance, but it is concerned with the complex mechanisms with which delinquency is controlled, pursued, punished and reformed." In the context of a society where communication is being pushed to the fore, the vocal delinquent will have more economic importance than would the criminal delinquent, yet Foucault's point stands. The technologies invented to curb the defective and reinforce class and race distinctions start to become economically and politically useful (101), which results in speech correction circulating more densely within the social field. However important immediate economic productivity may be, speech correction filled the much larger role of consolidating and maintaining a system of normalisation over subjects of speech.

I have argued that an articulate and fluent population is a historical biopolitical development, that the *dispositif* of speech correction—now termed speech-language pathology—emerges during the early twentieth century in order to make the capacity of speech manageable, efficient, and thus productive. This short history is obviously partial—riddled with holes and severed at both ends. (For a more complete tale, Daniel Martin's [2020] critical history of SLP in the Victorian era is excellent, as is Zara Richter's work [2020] on the classification and diagnosis of speech and its pathologies in the twentieth century.) Nevertheless, it serves the point I want to make: SLP is constitutive of a therapeutic regime consistent with liberal and neoliberal governmentality.

Despite being ostensibly mobilised to mitigate the social and economic threat of the speech defective, SLP has come to totalise the subject of speech. (Or, reading SLP as a colonial project to civilise speech, we can argue SLP has *colonised* the speaking subject.) For, unlike nineteenth-century attempts to correct speech, the twentieth-century *dispositif* was increasingly recognised as scientific (St. Pierre and St. Pierre 2018) and began to circulate within society via public and private school systems, child-guidance clinics, and hospital clinics during the 1920s and '30s—interpellating the normal subject of speech in its discipline of the abnormal. Since speech could not flow within productive channels until it had been made a docile object and capacity, speech correction should accordingly be understood as an *industry* that first renders speech intelligible as a biopolitical capacity whose insertion into the world (and capitalist machinery) *can* be regulated and controlled, and second, produces fluent semiotic subjects though a dense matrix of normalisation spread throughout institutions and social structures.

If SLP is an industry of the means of production that produces biopolitical subjects of speech, it does so in a largely implicit manner. Only a small percentage of the population have speech disabilities and will find themselves face-to-face with an SLP, although many more will interact with this *dispositif* in more diffuse ways. Yet this is not so different from many other contemporary apparatuses of power. The prison-industrial complex, for example, interpellates juridical subjects not through the constant threat of the sword, but through a panoptical gaze internalised by the population through popular media and a multitude of para-penal institutions. We participate in this form of subjection directly and indirectly, willing and not. Likewise, speech correction initiates a matrix of surveillance and self-surveillance that saturates the very capacity to speak, a condition of possibility of one's speech entering the world *as* speech, and thus, of oneself entering the world as a sufficiently human and political agent. The internalisation of the speech correctionist's gaze shapes our comportment to interlocutors, to the utterance, to language, and to authority in a manifold (and normalising) way. Our very communicative opening to the world is constituted by technologies of subjection that continually attempt to render communication a techne rather than an ethos. This matrix of speech correction enmeshes with and quickens other technologies of subjection, such as psychology, medicine, and of course, capitalism. Yet while suggestive, the argument that speech correction is an industry of the informational means of production is still missing an important and final step: namely, the leap from biopolitics to info-labour. I suggest that the discourse of "human capital" is the bridge between these two apparatuses. That is, human capital renders speech a depolitical and individual capacity that one *must* work on as a good neoliberal subject.

(Nonproductive) Human Capital

In *The Birth of Biopolitics*, Foucault, like David Harvey (2007), traces the concept of "human capital" to midtwentieth-century American neoliberals such as Gary Becker and Theodore Schultz. Whereas Marx identifies capital with wealth reinvested in production, and thus necessarily bound up with class relations, Becker and Schultz individualise and thereby depoliticise the concept. Foucault (2008) argues more specifically that neoliberals reorient "capital" from the perspective of the worker rather than the system. As he writes:

> [W]e will call "capital" everything that in one way or another can be a source of future income. Consequently, if we accept on this basis that the wage is an income, then the wage is therefore the income of a capital. Now what is the capital of which the wage is the income?

> Well, it is the set of all those physical and psychological factors which make someone able to earn this or that wage, so that, seen from the side of the worker, labour is not a commodity reduced by abstraction to labour power and the time [during] which it is used. (224)

From the worker's perspective, "capital" is that which will produce a return, a future income—a wage—such that labour is not a commodity sold to the bourgeoisie, but is a skill, an ability, or a form of capital. In this way, the capacities of the labouring subject become piecemeal sites of investment for future income—an enterprise (225). The discourse of human capital jettisons the responsibility for procuring an income (or being "successful" in any area of one's life) onto each individual subject, since the inability to earn an adequate wage can be read as a simple failure to plan for the future, a failure to invest properly in oneself as an enterprise.

The subject produced by and for neoliberalism—*homo economicus*—is a being emptied of political and civic capacities who only recognises and responds to the logic of the market. Neoliberalism enshrines the market (and its signals) as the singular source of truth and thereby consolidates its power over the subject by transforming every human action in every domain into economic terms. "Power," Foucault (252) writes, "gets a hold on [the neoliberal subject] to the extent, and only to the extent, that he is a *homo œconomicus*." Every subject and action must be evaluable in the financial terms of investment, risk, and return. Thus is *homo economicus* impelled to relate to itself as "human capital" and responsibly invest in its capacities to thereby increase its value in a global field of fierce competition and precarity.

The forces of neoliberalism and financialisation produce a new model of subjectivity: not, the theorist Michel Feher (2009) suggests, a liberal subject who *possesses* a capacity of labour-power apart from the essence of oneself, a capacity measurable in biological time that *belongs* to a subject and can thus be sold, but rather human capital that one can invest in but never sell. "As investors in their own human capital," Feher explains, "the subjects that are presupposed and targeted by neoliberalism can thus be conceived as the managers of a portfolio of conducts pertaining to all the aspects of their lives" (30). We can here recall the disabled participants of Butler's study who have accepted the need for straight talk as a condition for market, and by extension, for social value. The discourses of human capital and speech therapy here align: dysfluent speakers are taught to "manage" their (low-value) speech in the clinic. Speech therapy installs a panopticon inside each client, sending the subject into the world with technologies to self-police and regulate their dysfluent speech. In a profoundly alienating way, yet in perfect alignment with neoliberal practice, the logic of therapy renders the individual responsible at each moment for the value of their communicative capital—we neither own nor belong with our voices, but simply manage them.

Organising labour in terms of human capital enables neoliberalism to consolidate capital's grasp on the worker in a postindustrial age. Imagining the worker as a composite of various "capital-abilities" (Foucault 2008, 225) that must be invested in if one is to see return folds the production of communicative competence into the operations of capital while simultaneously making the subject solely responsible for its inevitable failure at compulsory able-bodiedness. This is the real subsumption of subjectivity, a site where Foucault and Marx meet. To become human capital, one must relate to oneself as a project through technologies of subjection. This is not an ethical project of relating to oneself, as Foucault (2003a; 2005) imagines in his later work, but a project or enterprise that serves the demands of capital and biopolitical governmentality. Becoming a fluent subject of speech is a crucial investment in one's human capital (an investment that makes future and ancillary investments possible), since, in part, the technology of fluency seeks to render human subjects governable and unambiguously representable within the apparatus of biopower.

Given enough time and accommodation, most people with speech disabilities can communicate. But simple information transfer itself is not where communicative capital gets mined. Paterson (2012, 166) suggests that "compliance with the notations of intercorporeal encounters has exchange value: it accords communicative capital." What matters most in environments like the workplace is the social dance of communication—the normalised gestures and temporal cues that render a speaker recognisable as a speaker. It is such that "[t]he choreography of communication has produced a context for embodied action in which people with speech impairment are framed as being 'out of time' and 'out of step' and so credited with little or no communicative capital" (2012, 166).

If one grows their portfolio of communicative capital by complying with social norms of communication, the language of "straight speech" is perhaps telling. Queer theorist Elizabeth Freeman (2010) offers the concept of "chrononormativity" to describe the organisation of temporal bodies toward optimal productivity. Chrononormative practices seek to eliminate temporal friction in productive domains while increasing it elsewhere: they "quicken up and/or synchronise some elements of everyday existence, while offering up other spaces and activities as leisurely, slow, sacred, cyclical, and so on and thereby repressing or effacing alternative strategies of organising time" (12). The unproductive time of queers and crips is a drag on progress. I have argued elsewhere (St. Pierre 2015) that choreographies of fluency are intertwined with unstable performances of masculinity and heteronormativity. The male stutterer disrupts a world ordered by normative time, what Kafer (2013, 34) calls "straight time," defined as "a firm delineation between past/present/future or an expectation of a linear development from dependent childhood to independent reproductive adulthood." In so doing he enters nonnormative time and thereby fumbles the social performance of masculinity. There is indeed a queerness in the inability to speak straight, one that threatens one's recognition as a full speaking subject who is unambiguously legible. As Butler (2014, 725) explains, "their level of fluency directly impacted on whether their message was heard and acted upon" by coworkers and customers alike. Dysfluency, by transgressing norms across the social field and desynchronising time, disqualifies a message qua message and a messenger qua messenger. Keeping in mind that this threat is experienced more complexly by people who live at multiple axes of oppression, dysfluency represents the erasure of a communicative subject and erosion of communicative capital.

The intersubjective choreographies that amplify the voices of some but discard others from the event of communication are inflected with distinctly social norms of classed, racialised, and gendered difference. However, as was already suggested by the "vocal smudge," and as I detail in the next chapter, there is a machinelike quality to proper speech that hides beneath its veil of social norms. "Progress is a forward march," writes Anna Lowenhaupt Tsing (2015, 21), "drawing other kinds of time into its rhythms. Without that driving beat, we might note other temporal patterns." The refusal of dysfluent bodies to keep step with capitalist time can help us notice differential temporal patterns—perhaps first that the expected pace of communication (that driving beat) keeps accelerating! Being "cast out of time" (Kafer 2013, 34) is a worry many disabled people face; for stutterers this fear is especially conditioned by our failure to become an instrument of acceleration. The dysfluent subject is unable to host capitalist time; we cannot facilitate the inhuman speeds demanded by the routines of semiotic labour.

In short, when conceived as human capital, speech becomes a private faculty that one manages but never owns. This transformation is profoundly alienating—for nondisabled voices, yes, but especially for disabled voices that are already estranged from dominant choreographies of communication. Speech as human capital moreover becomes a capacity that one *must* work on to subsist within info-capitalism; its future value relies on ongoing therapeutic maintenance that must ultimately be assumed by the individual as an individual.

Conclusion

The ableist choreographies of info-capitalism that attempt to shoot speech down straight lines are impossible in their compulsory and inhuman demands. Goodley (2014, xiv) writes that "[o]ur bodies are shaped by the alienating choreographies of capitalism. All of us are left lacking in the market; debilitated by the dance of capital." The dance of info-capitalism that keeps accelerating beyond human limits affects us all; it debilitates even nondisabled communicators (at least some of the time); it extracts information from body-minds and leaves them worn down. "We therefore," he continues, "need our interconnections, communities and alliances more than ever." The capitalisation of the voice subsumes its singularity, yet attending to those aspects of communication that refuse to be transformed by capital can sketch out a common site of politics and resistance.

To desire interconnection and community in critique of fluency is, of course, to invoke irony: connection in a hyperstimulated world is often the very problem for the dysfluent. Mitchell and Snyder (2010, 184) term "nonproductive bodies" those deemed "unfit" by capitalism. They "represent the non-laboring populations—not merely excluded from—but also resistant to standardized labor demands of human value." Like both Goodley and Sunaura Taylor, Mitchell and Snyder follow the line of flight produced by the excess of capitalism. The nonproductive bodies "whom Frantz Fanon designated 'the wretched of the earth' come into greater contact with each other through immaterial communication networks characteristic of modes of production in affective labor markets" (187). While Mitchell and Snyder are hopeful about new possibilities for collective action afforded by conditions of immaterial labour, this optimism must be tempered by an analysis of differential inclusion within immaterial and affective labour markets. We should ask, in other words: Does the valorisation of "contact" and "interconnection" establish or subvert new hierarchies of ability? Does it foreclose or open up new modes of communication and relation? Is access to communication networks "consumptive" or "transformative" (Brewer, Selfe, and Yergeau 2014)? Can we extend the nonproductive agency of living labour (the agency of Bartleby and nonproductive bodies) to subjectivities of communication? Can we imagine the trembled silence of stuttering as both refusal and invitation? Such questions are perhaps good starting points, but insufficient in themselves to muster any challenge to the logic of neoliberalism.

At stake is the capitalisation not just of "communication" but of relationality. Consider Richard, a civil servant interviewed by Butler, who illustrates the possibilities of dysfluent gain yet also its immediate capture. Although his boss complains that Richard's speech "upsets the flow of the meeting," Richard's critique of cheap talk is adamant: "But while they're talking they're missing so much. They miss what's not being said. They're so busy talking they miss the body language, the feel of meeting. Best bloody training for listening is having a stammer. . . . What is it financial, human and social capital? What about listening capital, does that exist? You should invent it" (726–27). This attunement to the world gained through a history of communicative marginalisation is a common refrain within dysfluent communities. But notice how quickly new possibilities for relationality collapse into capacities of human capital that are subservient to managerial ends. According to Butler, "the increased drive for verbal communication in the workplace was considered to be eradicating other ways of connecting" (727). How then might we cultivate forms of crip relationality that avoid immediate capture by therapeusis and neoliberal capital? How might we dwell within the refusal of fluency?

Learning to notice and learning to dwell within the slow and inarticulate can reorient our political intuitions. Recall the words of Brian cited in the opening vignette: "[t]here's more to work than talking straight isn't there? Some straight talkers talk rubbish but that's alright is it?" (2014, 724). The ableist imaginary takes the fluent voice as trustworthy and maps suspicion and risk upon the stutter (again, refracted through multiple axes of power). Yet with Brian, it seems clear that straight talk *is* so often a conduit for cheap talk—a pipeline for rubbish. And inversely, there *is* more to working than talking straight. "Each laborer," writes Goodley (2014, 94), "has the transformative and creative capacities of their labour to fashion alternative modes of production, consumption, and exchange." This is the excess of both living labour and neoliberalism that the latter needs but always struggles to control. The dysfluent refusal to match social norms of communication offers one possible site within which the value and meaning of speech—the *weight* of words (Campbell 2018)—can be reimagined. Perhaps having to wrestle and wait within the economy of words and meaning can offer a type of epistemic and political resource for communities of practice.

This reading of dysfluency, considered as a material agentic capacity, has already left the arena of cognitive capitalism, of the subject and language. This is perhaps for the best. Resisting the spell of the linguistic and info-capitalism requires that we find ways to exit the game of language and the strategies that impel us to play within the rules of intelligibility.

Two

Controlling Communication

This chapter turns from the domain of the human subject to examine how societies of control dissolve the social field and bodies themselves into an informational schema engaged in a universal struggle against noise. I argue that control over the process and act of communication via the filtering of unwanted and dangerous noise from mediums of communication relies on a depoliticisation of both noise and disability that renders communication inert. But in the final turn I suggest with Jane Bennett and Hasana Sharp that the tongue is ultimately uncontrollable—not governed by the will, but activated by proximate bodies in our world. Thus if dysfluency *is* a problem in information societies, it is not one of communication itself, but of control.

Vignette 5: Delayed Auditory Feedback (The SpeechEasy)

At seventeen I implored a charity and borrowed six thousand dollars from my grandma to invest the remainder of my hope in a cybernetic cure for stuttering. The SpeechEasy is a custom-fit earpiece marketed as "the world's smallest anti-stuttering device" (Janus Development Group, n.d.). A delayed auditory feedback device, the SpeechEasy delays and raises the pitch of one's voice to simulate the so-called "choral effect"—a well-known yet peculiar phenomenon where a stutterer's fluency dramatically increases while singing or speaking in unison with others. While the underlying science is still fuzzy, the SpeechEasy can "increase [one's] ability to communicate effectively and confidently" (Janus Development Group, n.d.) when the brain thinks the voice is not alone. Put simply, the SpeechEasy is a small, discrete device with a curative purpose—to make me stutter less and talk more. It is a feedback device that splits the voice to render it both output *and* input in an informational system. Under good conditions the device made my world sound squeaky, like a Chipmunks episode—but it could pull words from my lips in a steady stream, cleaning enough noise from my body to render it a relatively stable communication channel. Under bad conditions, I heard only overwhelming noise. In either case, it only "worked" for a year until my brain caught on to the trick and my stutter returned. The SpeechEasy landed in a dark drawer, but the financial debt lingered for years.

Vignette 6: Delayed Auditory Feedback (The SpeechJammer)

In 2012, two Japanese researchers, Kazutaka Kurihara and Koji Tsukada, published a report on a device called the SpeechJammer—a device that utilises delayed auditory feedback to create an effect opposite to that of the SpeechEasy: to *incapacitate* speaking by *producing* stuttering. While the researchers have no plans to market or develop their prototype further, the SpeechJammer resembles a clumsy toy gun and, with a directional microphone and speaker, returns a voice to the sender with a slight delay. This effectively jams the tongue, invoking automatic and uncontrollable stuttering. In the words of its creators, it jams "unimpaired people's speech whether they want it or not" (3). It is revealing that despite these opposite purposes, both the SpeechEasy and SpeechJammer are positioned as cures for informational maladies.

Kurihara and Tsukada suggest that the SpeechJammer can be used to create the conditions of rational deliberation, silencing interlocutors who speak out of turn, for example. "We live in the twenty-first century," write Kurihara and Tsukada, "when it is said that communication is the most important means of resolving conflicts. However, there are still many cases in which the negative aspects of speech become a barrier to the peaceful resolution of conflicts, sometimes further harming society" (1). Two accidental features of speech—or *negative* aspects—crop up: unavoidability and occupancy. As Kurihara and Tsukada explain, a listener can neither avoid speech once it has been sent into the world, nor can the human attention load handle more than two speakers at once. The SpeechJammer minimizes these negative characteristics of speech that, they argue, impede the goal of "peaceful communication" (4).

Kurihara and Tsukada thus offer in the SpeechJammer a *technical fix* for a long-standing democratic problem: How do we establish and enforce rational norms of deliberation in order to resolve conflict and reach agreement? How do we safeguard against might (loud and fluent voices) equaling right? The SpeechJammer short-circuits such troublesome questions that define political practice. It brings a feedback gun to a word conflict; it establishes communicative norms by force! There is a clear echo of Mao Zedong (1972, 61) in the silence of stopped tongues: "Political power grows out of the barrel of a gun." Whether or not they materialise, the possible uses of this faux-Habermasian gift are chilling.[1]

• • •

One consistent feature of biopolitical techniques is their naturalisation of biological difference. The management of populations and individuals hides the *historically specific* processes of creating and sorting difference under banners of transhistorical universality. Disability, we are asked to believe, *simply is*: an unchanging fact of human bodies and scientific inquiry. I have been told with patronising smiles that both the etiology and treatment of stuttering are best left in the hands of "experts." In the last chapter I suggested that the therapeutic regime of speech-language pathology naturalises dys/fluency; here I add midcentury cybernetics and information theory to the mix as a second source of authority over the communicative body. Like SLP, information theory reduces the event of communication to a technical and thus optimisable process from beginning to end. And like SLP, information theory trades in noisy bodies.

We could trace a longer history across Western thought of the partition made between those who speak rationally, and thus belong to the polis, and "barbarians"—outsiders who, literally, can merely babble. Walling off rational communities of speech from noise through a coding of the social body is a thoroughly political act, and one, I would guess, that has existed in a nearly unbroken sequence down through Western history. Nevertheless, cybernetics revolutionised this project by joining under one banner "communication" and "control." Cybernetics is the science of control, defined in 1950 by Norbert Wiener as the scientific study of "control and communication in the animal and the machine"; this popular discipline sought to recode the universe in terms of information exchange and homeostatic systems, and to exercise control over the human and its environment through these means.

Cybernetics is in this way a cutting edge that enacts a series of deterritorialisations in the social field. Wiener and his followers conceive of the human and society itself in terms of information flow (the organism being a vast network of genetic and molecular codes), which makes protecting this flow from dissipation—whether from external force or internal corruption—a moral activity. As Wiener (1950, 131) proclaimed during the Cold War, "The integrity of the channels of internal communication is essential to the welfare of society." Liberalism champions free information to procure it as an essential recourse. In turn, entropic forces such as dysfluency (and deafness, on which

Wiener fixated) degrade the integrity of the channel and thus impede the free flow of communication, making it not merely a technical problem, but a social and even existential risk.

Cybernetics formalised communication into the process of *transmitting messages*, a process best understood as a game played by interlocutors against the third party of noise. Noise here corresponds to entropy, the decay of informational patterns into disorganisation. Feedback, in turn, is a regulatory mechanism that both reduces noise in a system and controls its states—for example, commanding a satellite to reposition. Defining the boundaries of a channel precedes transmitting messages, and, explains Kai Eriksson (2008, 280–81), it is such that "the pursuit of a common code, form, or method, has characterised the modern history of communication. This protected meaningful communication from misunderstanding and interference." In this context, a code describes a formalised alliance against noise, one not restricted to information and communication technologies but also manifest in embodied choreographies of communication. Habituated expectations of what sort of speech is appropriate and useful within given contexts solidify into unspoken communicative rules embedded in the social fabric, rules that exclude certain voices and behaviours as disorganising forces.

The SpeechEasy and SpeechJammer are thus cybernetic devices not because of their size or, strictly speaking, technology, but because as interfaces they render their users part of an informational system defined by a universal struggle against noise. The feedback technology of the SpeechEasy is crude, since it basically jams a single modulation into the brain and hopes for the best. Yet we can nevertheless examine the functions of such machines. What do they *do*? The outputs of SpeechEasy and SpeechJammer may differ—one seems to cure dysfluency and the other to produce it—but they share the fantasy of controlling the tongue.

Several nested operations are presupposed and enacted by the SpeechEasy and SpeechJammer. They first render noise a universal and *apolitical* enemy; second, they figure dysfluency as noise; and third, they clean noise from public media (that together form a market). Since, Kurihara and Tsukada argue, speech "cannot be easily avoided by listeners, we have established a consensus that we should not generate excessive levels of noise in public" (1). I concede that noise pollution such as aircraft engines or loud music seeps unwanted into aural spaces, and also that this phenomenon is underwritten by the sense of hearing, which is uniquely exposed to the world. Yet what Kurihara and Tsukada offer is more: an abstraction that disavows its own political conditions. To claim "we have established a consensus . . ." invokes a system of compulsory able-bodiedness (McRuer 2006) that assumes an apparent consensus on the undesirability of disability. "That we should not generate excessive levels of noise in public" relitigates Susan Schweik's (2009) study of the nineteenth-century "ugly laws" in the US that excluded unsightly bodies from public visibility. In this way, to reference *excess* levels of noise is a matter of quality as much as quantity: What sorts of voices do we consider undesirable? What sorts of voices do we filter from sonic public space? Kurihara and Tsukada openly equate dysfluent voices with noise pollution—an unwanted and disorganising force—that has no place in the public. The act of turning fluent voices dysfluent is the main event, for once the SpeechJammer has disabled a voice, cleaning noise from the public sphere and from rational deliberation is almost an afterthought.

Within the logic of information theory, the exclusion of nonuniversal embodiments makes sense. Compulsory able-bodiedness codes desire at a prepersonal level; it clears, through a process of standardisation that excludes "incommunicable" modes of expression and signification, a homogenous zone or *commons* within which to communicate. The problem of noisy, incommunicable bodies in social and political channels is thus not new, but nevertheless it became in the mid-twentieth century a *generalised* problematic of biopolitics. As Haraway explains (1990, 34), "Communications sciences and modern biologies are constructed by a common move—*the translation of the world into a problem of coding*, a search for a common language in which all resistance to instrumental control disappears" (emphasis in original). Starting with cybernetics, then endocrinology, and flourishing in the '70s with pharmacology, immunology, systems theory, and neo-Darwinist genetics (both population and molecular), the biological and communications sciences have entangled themselves in a common project and common language. It should thus not surprise us to find information sciences and neo-eugenics together in bed.[2] Both projects decode life into a form pliable to instrumental control and optimisation—an alliance that Virilio (1999, 132) calls "cybernetic eugenicism."

Haraway notes that the modern creation of information has made possible (if never fully attainable) a universal code that enables universal translation between heterogeneous elements, and thus universal control. Unhindered communication is essential for these operations, yet boundaries are not equally permeable to information. Indeed, "[t]he biggest threat to such power is interruption of communication. Any system breakdown is a function of stress" (34). Feedback machines that purge bodies of noise offer one fix. Yet on a macro level, the control of heterogeneous bodies of information requires more complex techniques of risk analysis that differentially assess and filter flows.

Risk and Control

Vignette 7: Stuttering through Security

On January 21, 2017, Kylie Simmons, a Black US citizen, returned to the US after studying in Costa Rica for six months. However, she was detained in Hartsfield-Jackson Atlanta International Airport after she stuttered on the first question by Customs and Border Protection: from what country did you come? The stutter raised suspicion. Simmons was immediately detained and asked humiliating questions, even, she (2016) recounts, about whether she even *did* stutter "because the staffer said that I was not stuttering when speaking with him." She was called dishonest and she missed her connecting flight, but Simmons gained national and international attention with the social media campaign #DDDetainedInAtlanta. This prompted an apology from Customs and Border Protection and a commitment to develop training resources for their officers about people who stutter.

Vignette 8: Vocal Risk Assessment

The California-based start-up Clearspeed™ quantifies the risk that individuals pose to a system based solely on *how* they speak. Interviewees respond "yes" or "no" to simple questions and the machine learning behind Remote Risk Assessment (RRA®) uses "unique voice analytic processes to evaluate and quantify distinct characteristics of the human voice related to risk" such as pitch, speed, and hesitancy. This technology can be used to screen migrants at borders, current employees for corporate espionage, or insurance applicants for fraud. The *old* tagline for the technology read, "We accelerate the speed of trust." The new one tries a different, yet no less ominous, approach: "Using the power of voice for good."

• • •

What Simmons was made to endure reveals the mechanisms by which a "society of control," a concept popularised by Deleuze in 1992, regulates the flow of informational bodies. Built from the technological and social architecture of cybernetics (and infused with speculative capital), societies of control govern system components within an open field. Rather than patterning bodies with a uniform cast (the worker, the prisoner, the student, the normate), societies of control modulate the capacities of the body for localised needs. "No objects, spaces, or bodies are sacred in themselves" (Haraway 1990, 32). Instead of containing bodies within discontinuous spaces such as the factory, the prison, the school, or the institution, control marshalls credit or risk scores that travel anywhere. The bounded factory gives way to the corporate ladder and the mobile office—the entrepreneur-on-the-go. The prison-industrial complex expands through technologies of geo-tagged parole. The school opens to online learning, lifelong learning, and professional development. Within societies of control, Deleuze insists, one never arrives. Moreover, each deterritorialisation renders the user "free" to move within a social field and adapts to their schedule, yet always at the cost of information: the throughput of postindustrial machines that control societies ruthlessly extract from human and nonhuman bodies.

Control manages where and how fast flows can pass, positively channelling potentialities. This means that we are, ostensibly, free to express ourselves on social media and free to work abroad or from home, but always on infinitely expanding highways of information where each move that constitutes our digital profile is carefully tracked, packaged, and sold by big data. Deleuze (2006, 322) writes: "You do not confine people with a highway. But by making highways, you multiply the means of control. I am not saying this is the only aim of highways, but people can travel infinitely and 'freely' without being confined while being perfectly controlled. That is our future." So-called information highways likewise expand our possible communicative routes and horizons always within the parameters of control. And in turn, this smooth traffic of information increases the potential for both semiotic gridlocks and accidents.

Deleuze (1992, 5) explains that "the numerical language of control is made of codes that mark access to information or reject it." By code, Deleuze has in mind the predetermined codes that computers run, and especially the more flexible codes of DNA. And, as for Kylie Simmons, the notion of *access* (familiar to disability theory) describes the way we can move—or are blocked—within societies of control. The social field is here much like the internet: it offers the appearance of openness and continuousness, yet is constructed by protocols that can cause constrictions for any individual at any point. Sarah Sharma (2014) explains that for subjects imbued with enough biopolitical value, the world unfolds as "borderless" or "flat"—one can travel nearly anywhere with seemingly effortless speed. (As I explain below, this speed is always predicated on temporal maintenance performed by others.)

Yet, with the inhuman decision of an algorithm or the flick of a few keystrokes around the world, the numerical code scanned on one's passport or credit card can also revoke access to information, capital, or movement. Here the instrumental conceit of "universal communication" is clear—it depicts not universal access (to information or space) but the state of being *universally accessible* to control. "Controls are a *modulation*," writes Deleuze (1992, 4), "[l]ike a sieve whose mesh will transmute from point to point." If control societies are defined not by their boundaries but their operations on flows, the airport is perhaps a quintessential institution.

An airport is a "transit zone" within a nation's sovereign territory; an input-output terminal; an interface of flows of material, information, capital, the military, and migrants. I agree with Sharma (2014, 30) when she writes that "the importance of the airport has less to do with how it fails as a public space . . . and more to do with the way it operates within the larger biopolitical economy of time." At such points of crossing, the assessment of *risk* becomes a basic operation: who/what do we trust to pass and circulate where, when, and how fast? There is thus something terribly mundane about detaining Simmons for stuttering. In a typical day during 2017, the US Customs and Border Protection (2018) processed 340,444 international air passengers as they hunted for signals of risk. It is thus not merely numerical codes but also *social* codes that restrict access to flow. It matters that Simmons is Black in the US, where Black people are 5.9 times more likely to be incarcerated than white people. The uncertainty aroused by Simmons's stutter (*Why is she nervous? What is she hiding? What* risk *does she pose?*) and the disbelief about the very existence of her stutter are here inseparable from the cultural suspicion surrounding Black bodies. Simmons was rendered suspicious and dishonest through systems of compulsory fluency and white supremacy that are connected, as I argued in the last chapter, by a history of speech correction; together these systems mark the normate citizen subject (white and able-bodied) who can—and indeed, expects to—speed across borders with ease.

The type of intersectional discrimination that Simmons endured due to social coding is precisely what companies like Clearspeed (formerly AC Global Risk) claim to eliminate, for, according to the priests of Silicon Valley, the problems with screening lie in social bias and human inefficiency. The algorithms behind Remote Risk Assessment thus function to decode the voice: to scrape its *surface* for nervous tics, inflections, pauses, or intonations and then recompose its essence—with a highly accurate and scalable system. By registering the truth of self through the truth of the voice, or again, by investing in the voice as an empirical vehicle of truth-telling, risk-assessment algorithms seek to bypass the register of subjective *content* and thus the capacity to lie and be lied to.

This tagline—"We accelerate the speed of trust"—is not merely corporate marketing, but axiomatic of control. Analogous to Deleuze's analysis of control, what Foucault (2007) calls "security" is the governance of flows. These techniques, present already in eighteenth-century city planning, are a matter of "organizing circulation, eliminating its dangerous elements, making a division between good and bad circulation, and maximizing the good circulation by diminishing the bad" (18). The importance of categorising risk groups and maintaining differential rates for high- and low-risk bodies puts pressure on technologies of risk assessment to filter, with maximal accuracy and speed, the bad circulation from the good. The "speed of trust" thus marks a functional limit to the circulation of desirable flow. The acceleration of trust via a doubling down on boundary maintenance is, in turn, an axiomatic, basic command of control. This is especially true for the flow of information since, as Haraway reminds us, interruption to this particular flow results in stress on instrumental control. By recoding the voice as an informational surface that is legible to machines, Clearspeed purports to accelerate the *organisation* of circulation (to connect and disconnect flows ever faster). But how, we might wonder, would the algorithms that drive Remote Risk Assessment decode the voice of Simmons?

Considered together, this second pair of vignettes highlights how the information machines forged by cybernetics recode social practices and break down constitutive boundaries of the subject and human, reinscribing oppression for "high-risk" bodies on a machinic plane. Such changes indicate a larger shift in the governance of disability under neoliberalism. For Jasbir Puar (2013), the deterritorialising effects of information in forms such as surveillance and bioinformatic technologies have prompted new questions about the boundaries of life, and, moreover, a new mode of governing embodied difference. Instead of "regulating normativity," by which Puar means the imposition of a hegemonic norm on an entire population that cleaves the normal from the pathological, neoliberalism "regularises bodies." That is, neoliberalism modulates rather than moulds bodies, evaluating *all* "in relation to their success or failure in terms of health, wealth, progressive productivity, upward mobility, [and] enhanced capacity" (182). Instead of marking discrete kinds of being—a *normal* versus *pathological* organism or subject—capacity and debility index the gradated power of an assemblage; they are fluid biopolitical sites in which we can and must invest. Puar offers the example of mental health and argues that the surge of depression in the twenty-first century is the result of differential inclusion: not interpellating an increasing number of depressed subjects but asking "To what *degree* is one depressed?" (182; emphasis mine). The medical-industrial complex thus captures and activates modular components of the body (and population) that always have a statistical existence through which risk and prognosis can be calculated.

In a society of control, one is always in transit and never really finished with tasks such as work or school. Similarly, control submits the body to a continual process of optimisation such that, as Puar writes, "[t]here is no such thing as an 'adequately abled' body anymore" (182). Neoliberalism decodes social practices that once afforded local function and value to bodily capacities in order to submit the flow of bodies to its simple axiom: "Connect those flows! Faster, faster!" (Smith and Protevi 2018). An axiomatic is a command that, by nature, has no ground and thus no limit. When *no one* is adequately abled, then lifelong learning, professional development, rehabilitation, therapy (of all stripes), cosmetic surgery, diet, exercise, prosthetics, medical and student debt, and even doping all become ongoing imperatives to adjust one's risk value and become competitive as little bundles of capital.

Understood from its speculative logic, neoliberalism tears communication from its relations, material infrastructures, and networks of power to be rendered a distinctly *in*human ability into which one must invest continually and early.[3] SLP reads early childhood intervention as a site to invest in its capital by standardising the child's informatic future. Wearable devices are getting in on this action. In 2016, VersaMe, the now-defunct Silicon Valley start-up (the epitome of fast capitalism) launched a wearable device called "Starling." Clipped to an infant's clothing, Starling hid a microphone and counted the words spoken to and by the baby each day. Leveraging the premise that the more words a baby is exposed to—the more verbose the parents—the better the child's neurological development will be, parents were encouraged to set targets on the app and position even "nonsymptomatic" preverbal children as already in need of therapeutic intervention. As Wendy Brown (2015) argues, parental anxiety around the most minor lisp or "delayed development" in speech (and their own speech as para-practitioner parents!) is justified once the polity is laid bare to the fluctuations of macroeconomic growth. "As human capital, they may contribute to or be a drag on economic growth; they may be invested in or divested from depending on their potential for GDP enhancement" (110). The utter disposability of citizens under neoliberalism makes investment in "human" capital a grotesque moral obligation. This is particularly true for those coded as disabled, born a mishmash of high-risk profiles in a financialised and speculative world. Thus, despite the desedimentation of categories signalled by "debility," it is important to note that in a Venn diagram, "disabled" and "debilitated" bodies overlap significantly.

Information Machines

To appreciate how control societies capture the event of communication, we must understand two common yet enigmatic concepts: the machine and information.

First, with Guattari, it is important to note that the machine is not equivalent to the technical device. Guattari (1995a, 33) inverts the common-sense relation between the machine and technology such that "[t]he machine would become the prerequisite for technology rather than its expression." The technical machine, which runs on information and energy, is a *type* of machine, but itself only functions through its connections with other machines in which it is a component part. Guattari (1995b, 8) argues that reducing the machine to its materiality obscures its *ontogenetic* elements: those "elements of the plan, of construction, social relationships which support these technologies, a stock of knowledge, economic relations and a whole series of interfaces onto which the technical object attaches itself." The technical device is inseparable from its ontogenetic process. Yet the technological machine also sits within a machinic phylum—that is, within a lineage of machines that we can trace from Charles Babbage, the Jacquard loom, onwards.

The machine operates by a fundamental logic of connection: it forms linkages or "concatenations" between once-heterogeneous components. Open to the exterior, machines govern a field of always-changing *possible* relations and *virtual* connections such that, as Levi Bryant (2014, 40) explains, "the being of a machine is defined not by its qualities or properties, but rather by the operations of which it is capable." He suggests the question to ask is not "What are its properties?" but "What is a machine connected to? What operations does it perform? What does it make possible?" The machine is by definition an assemblage that includes technical aspects—what we typically mean by a machine—but also corporeal, social, intellectual, and semiotic organs. Because the machine is ontologically open to connection and thus to becoming, it can also lose its operational form. Machines creak and break. A speaking body can cross a limit-threshold where it is too dysfluent or slow or awkward to operate as a component part in a functional assemblage like a working group that follows corporate protocols and targets. But, as open assemblages, machines also repair/regenerate in unanticipated ways.

For example, in "A Manifesto for the Broken Machine," Sharma (2020) invites us to consider gender relations from inside a machinic logic. When techno-patriarchy reduces women to their functions (a home keeper, a reproduction unit, a sex receptacle), what are feminists—quips Sharma—but tools that have lost their use, vacuums that no longer suck? As such, "the imagined technological future is one in which social justice is no longer demanded because all of the seemingly malfunctioning parts (nonconforming subjects) can be discarded and replaced" (173). Rewriting the micropolitics of social oppression in machinic terms, Sharma suggests, for instance, that most forms of "representation" of "diverse" heads on panels or boardrooms are little more than *file retrieval*: people become data that can be pulled out when needed, then filed away. Yet despite the ways that the piles of Broken Machines produced by societies of control signal a technological landscape designed to subtend rather than question pre-existing structures of power, Sharma finds courage in the power-from-below of Broken Machines that refuse to function as designed. The #MeToo movement, for example, "revealed that perpetrators of sexual violence didn't think their women—as machines in relatively good working order—would talk among themselves or turn against them" (175). Docile components are designed to talk at work but surely never against their masters! That such machines would—could—form a new refrain to connect in unexpected ways was beyond the master's imagination.

Second, what of information? Like "machine," "information" is a common term that, in its modern usage, has a technical root and is thus also embedded in a machinic phylum. In the mid-twentieth century, Claude Shannon, a mathematician and engineer working at Bell Telephone Laboratories, distilled information down to a quantitative meaning: the statistical measure of uncertainty within a tightly defined system. He defined the "bit" as the basic unit of measurement, "the smallest possible quantity of information [that] represents the amount of uncertainty that exists in the flipping of a coin" (Gleick 238). Constructed within a schema of pattern/randomness, greater uncertainty equals more information. A greater improbability of a state (that, for example, 'u' does not follow 'q') corresponds to more information sent. It is such that the amount of information in a sentence can be calculated (in bites) and the *transmission* of information optimised. Insofar as the goal of information theory is the *efficient* and *invariant* transmission of information across heterogeneous milieus (Lazzarato 2014, 72), communication becomes a problem of entropy: the tendency of a system to become disorganised; of a signal to dissipate in transmission; of contact to collapse back into noise.

It is significant that Shannon was employed at Bell Labs when he sparked the information revolution. One reason it is significant is that it locates modern information within what James Carey (2008, 13) calls the "transmission model" of communication: the imperial notion that "communication is a process whereby messages are transmitted and distributed in space for the control of distance and people." Another is that it places Shannon within a lineage of people and processes committed to stamping out noise with moral authority. I return to both of these issues below.

Tiziana Terranova (2004) explains the concept of information by peeling apart two different registers and logics.[4] In its most common sense, information is representational. This refers to the semantic content of a message and its meaning—to *signs*. But at a more basic level, information refers to *signals*: the material impulses defined against noise that carry a message through a channel. Terranova argues that the fundamental informatic problematic is how to establish the minimum conditions for *contact* between sender and receiver. As we already witnessed with the SpeechEasy and SpeechJammer, contact implies a type of alliance created between a sender and receiver against the third party of noise. "Speech is a joint game by the talker and the listener against the forces of confusion" (Wiener 1950, 92). "Successful" communication is first and foremost not an interpretive but an operational game, such that information theory ascribes "*secondary* importance to the question of the *meaning* of messages when compared to the basic problem of *how to increase the effectiveness of the channel*" (Terranova 14; emphasis in original). The distinctly inhuman force of noise becomes the universal enemy—shifting the register of communication politics from subjective to machinic.

These two regimes of sign and signal were present at the founding of information theory. While cybernetics did not survive the '60s, its spirit endured in the formal theories it generated regarding information, communication, systems, and control. In 1963, Claude Shannon and Warren Weaver defined communication as the "procedures by which one mind [or mechanism] may affect another" (3). More specifically, Shannon and Weaver problematise communication at three registers:

1. The *technical* problem—"How accurately can the symbols of communication be transmitted?"
2. The *semantic* or *philosophical* problem—"How precisely do the transmitted symbols convey the desired meaning?"
3. The *effectiveness problem*—"How effectively does the received meaning affect conduct in the desired way?" (4)

This set of conceptual and technical problems revolves around accurately transmitting a message across a noisy medium. It is such that communication theorists use language such as the "transmission model" or the "conduit metaphor" (Reddy 1979), where as Ronald Day (2001, 41) explains, information is considered the encoded flow of a message from one source to another. This process entails (1) the subjective intention of a message, (2) encoded and transmitted across a clear medium such that this intention can be (3) reproduced in the mind of the other, (4) the accuracy of which is measured by behavioural effects. For cybernetics the final step is (5) feeding information back into the system to control its states.

Problems of meaning are here, again, secondary to problems of noise. It is helpful to consider the production of noiseless channels from the perspective of disability history. Deaf scholars are uniquely attuned to the materiality of information technologies, the embodied mediums through which information travels. Mara Mills (2011, 83), a historian of disability and media, argues (*pace* Hayles 1999) that cybernetics did not seek to abstract information from materiality, but was deeply invested in the body—specifically in the policing of human difference—to produce smooth forms of (bio)media that carry signals efficiently. While Mills is most concerned with the intertwined development of deaf education and communication engineering, in her analysis speech is never far off. This makes sense insofar as deafness is constructed within an environment of strident oralism. Specifically, she argues that information engineers and theorists took as their model face-to-face oral conversation, assuming that speech (rather than writing or sign) was most informationally efficient and best conveyed the intentions of the sender.[5]

The goal of invariant information transmission requires by necessity a hypernormalised social body. Mills argues that hard-of-hearing activists were well aware that clear channels (voices) were required to be included in the communication society. She cites the midcentury activist Florence Hazzard:

> We underhearing people are apt to forget what a strong influence sound has on the emotions. . . . And the effects our voices have on our normal hearing friends are too frequently boredom (from lack of color and inflection), fatigue (from straining to hear a low mumble-mumble), annoyance (from the nervous shock of being shouted at). (cited in Mills 87)

Uncommon pronunciation (the so-called deaf accent) impedes the invariant transfer of information at the affective and signifying register. It affects and *demands* something from the listener—and thus widens the aperture of the encounter beyond functional limits. Much like the dysfluent voice, the discomfort of the deaf voice slows down the sensible process of interpretation and frames such mediums as inefficient carriers of information. Wiener agrees. "The vast majority of deaf mutes," he wrote in 1949, "though they can learn how to use their lips and mouths to produce sound, do so with a grotesque and harsh intonation, which represents a highly inefficient form of sending a message" (260). The affectivity of the deaf voice must be normalised to constitute a stable communication channel. As Mills writes, "[t]he ideal, which affected both human and machine communication, was universal, frictionless, instantaneous, and economical" (87). Put otherwise, and as I will explore further in the next chapter, "inclusion" into mainstream communication flows and into the public itself hinges on disabled and other minor voices conforming to such operational norms.

Because sending a message requires keeping figure and ground separate, Day (2001, 33) notes that the task for communication sciences is to adjudicate "desirable uncertainty" from "undesirable uncertainty." Good uncertainty refers to the sender's freedom to choose one message over another, while bad uncertainty is "uncertainty which arises because of errors or because of the influence of noise" (Shannon and Weaver 1963, 19). Good uncertainty can be statistically defined and is foregrounded against chaotic uncertainty, the static we take to be "irrelevant noise" but that nevertheless seeps into channels and confuses not only the boundaries of the system but the agency (the good freedom) of the communicative agents.

Although formalised by information theory, liberalism has from the start conceived of communication as exchange, as a problem, and has erased disability in its pursuit of the universal. John Durham Peters (1989) traces Locke's contribution to the transmission model of communication, understood here as the process of transmitting ideas between minds with words. As Peters explains, a type of "linguistic individualism" infuses Locke's political theory insofar as meaning is necessarily private: it corresponds to ideas inside the mind rather than either referents in the world or a semiotic system (391). The communicative event within the liberal imaginary is thus constituted by two poles (sender and receiver) that are separated by the ontological chasm of private/public, interior-/exterior. This makes communication a dilemma—miscommunication and confusion will occur without symmetry between the sender-idea and receiver-idea. The walls erected around the private sphere thus present a troubling existential and linguistic problem for Locke. "[T]he individual (and not society, language, or tradition) is the master of meaning, which makes common understanding between individuals both desperately urgent and highly problematic" (389). If communication as *common* meaning becomes both necessary and impossible, how do we know that we are genuinely communicating with others? How can civil society be constructed and sustained under such conditions?

Peters highlights the etymological root of communication as transmission: transporting commercial goods. The risk in both of these ventures lies in protecting the integrity of the message or commodity from interference during its voyage into the public sphere. Just as the quantity and quality of wheat sent must match what is received, so for communication to be successful the idea sent must be identical to that received. As "a utilitarian device for sending clear ideas and avoiding confusion" (391), communication becomes a distinctly technical and political problematic. The interiority of meaning renders the public sphere (the market), and the material signs that must venture into its domain, threats to liberal capitalism, threats that must constantly be surveilled and managed. Moreover, liberal capitalism must ward against the *intentional* interference of agents who would steal, corrupt, or otherwise infiltrate an exchange. Thus do communication technologies encode messages to evade enemy interception, and thus does the integrity or *trustworthiness* of the channel become a technical matter to maintain. As Clearspeed explains very plainly: "Our vision is to help build a safer world through trust enablement" (n.d.).

The conduit metaphor adopts and retains this basic Lockean problematic. It presumes the freedom of the individual sender, the equality of exchange, the danger of public mediums and the need to keep them clear, the commodification of signs, the frailty of the message, and thus the necessity of both security and the contractual, formalised relation. Yet information theory also translates these problems into a more deterritorialised form representable in the neutral terms of systems theory. It transforms the public/private divide, which excludes disabled subjects from the political sphere of rational discourse, into the operational (and far cleaner) distinction between system and noise. In this way, explains Day (2001, 43), Shannon and Weaver reduce "all anomalies or alterities of representation to 'abnormal' statistical appearances within the range of a normative communication system." Dysfluency cannot be excluded from the political when the political does not exist.

Moreover, information theory resolves the liberal aporia of communication through feedback. Wiener, Shannon, and Weaver alike flatten the communicative assemblage into purely operational relations that focus on definitive and behaviouristic outcomes. Understanding—at least enough for functional communication—is confirmed by the observation of behavioural effects: the exchange of information triggers cycles of action and reaction recognisable by informational systems. This move by information theory, writes Day, "reduces all affective events to being *effective* events (thus requiring an intentional or causal subject-object relationship and introducing issues of probability, measurement, noise and delay, and feedback)" (41). The grammar of control de-animates the body of communication by reducing its action to causal behaviour.[6] In doing so, it safeguards the liberal freedom of speaker and listener, but also enables fleshy bodies of communication to accelerate in order to match the inhuman beat of capital.

The Speed of Contact

The sociologist John Tomlinson (2007) reads the modern narrative of progressive enlightenment as a tale of overcoming the limits of nature through speed, and makes a helpful distinction among several modes of speed: first, "machine speed" ordered by an instrumental rationality; second, the "unruly speed" of, for example, the sportscar that fuels and is fuelled by liberal desires for individual freedom, risk, and euphoria; and third, what Tomlinson calls a "condition of immediacy." I will set unruly speed to the side in this particular discussion, while recognising that a form of "speed heroism" (52) that attaches to unruly speed does condition the desire to accelerate straight speech.

Machine or *mechanical* speed seeks to overcome "the 'natural' resistance of physical space to the fulfillment of human desire" (78). Thermodynamic machines such as the railway that exceeded the ostensibly natural limitations of the body and materiality itself collapsed the gap between departure and arrival, "now from later, here from elsewhere, desire from its satisfaction" (74). There are, however, limits to the capacity of thermodynamic machines—laden with inertia and plagued by entropy—to close this gap. It is such that Tomlinson reads the midcentury information revolution as an accelerating force with both quantitative and qualitative effects. On the one hand, substituting objects (and persons) with information has produced possibilities for unbridled speed. Stocks, for example, are now traded by algorithms at a scale approaching nanoseconds. This speed far eclipses the human register and demands the use of machines to think, judge, and communicate in our stead.

More than this, the fact that we happily plug ourselves into human-machine assemblages, the fact that we so eagerly *desire* to share communicative agency with machines, speaks to the qualitative change their speed affords: immediacy is fundamentally a condition of *effortlessness*. Tomlinson reminds us that the concept tracks in both spatial and temporal registers: immediacy is proximity, or contact without mediation as well as instantaneity. Communication technologies slake my desire to connect with friends or colleagues worldwide. With a few twitches of my finger, we become talking heads "face-to-face" with seemingly nothing in between—if everything works. But somewhat like standards of female beauty that demand perfection (smooth lines and smooth skin) without a trace of the effort involved, the condition of immediacy must *deny* any mediation in order to seal the gap between departure and arrival.

Immediacy is a normative rather than descriptive claim about the world; it describes what we believe *ought* to be rather than what is. We believe communication ought to be controlled and rendered immediate, even though dropped calls, 404 errors, stuttered Zoom calls, and accidentally muted microphones are a mundane reality. Virilio and Lotringer (2002, 78) lament that in an information society "[w]e're no longer communicating. Communication itself is communicated without leaving a trace." But this too is an abstraction. It is such that immediacy, Tomlinson notes, requires an act of social imagination—to *believe* the gap is already closed and to make the middle term redundant (91). It is not merely dropped calls and long flights that must be forgotten: dysfluent and otherwise impure bodies must be purged from our mediums in order to reproduce the fantasy of effortless, instant speed.

Despite the fact that the plurality of bodies-in-time is always the stage on which communication plays, information sciences must standardise the communicative exchange towards the goal of a universal code—this is the only way to abstract from the co-mingled shit of bodies and construct highways that can approach a condition of immediacy. Put otherwise, information societies must *de-animate* the middle term to make belief in unmediated contact possible. De-animation occurs, as I explained above, when communication collapses into effective events that follow a logic of risk and speculation. There is here no *listening* but merely predicting in relation to a normative grammar. But de-animation is also presumed in the fantasy of docile communicative bodies. "Standardisation" is itself an abstraction that facilitates belief by hiding the violence needed to de-animate embodied mediums of communication.

Consider the figure of Alexander Graham Bell, who embodies two great projects of the late nineteenth century: eugenics and telecommunications. A staunch supporter of the "oralist" position, which (in counterdistinction to the "manualist" position) held that deaf people must be taught to speak rather than sign, Bell believed that the value of speech was beyond measure. If one *were* to appraise speech, Bell (1877, 178) opined, "we must not measure the value of speech by its *perfection*, but by its *intelligibility*. What is the object of the education of the deaf and dumb, if it is not to set them in communication with the world?" (emphasis added). Evaluating speech not by its perfection but by its intelligibility references the machinic problem of contact. Unlike the "perfect" speech of the bourgeoisie that marks and individuates a subject, the "intelligible" voice is thoroughly functional. The technical-philosophical dream of connecting the world through telephone wires, as well as the contiguous hurdles of entropy and interference, are mirrored in deaf and dysfluent bodies.[7] For Bell, the principal object of deaf education is to produce smooth surfaces of contact. Setting the deaf (and dysfluent) in "communication with the world" is thus thinly veiled language for assimilation and the erasure of semiotic difference. Bell was heavily invested in the eugenics movement, and while he did not advocate sterilisation, he did encourage the "evolution of a higher and nobler type of man in America" through legislative and educative means (1908, 214). Equally eugenic is his belief that deaf people should be assimilated into mainstream society to erase all cultural traces of deafness.

Shannon and Weaver define information as good uncertainty protected from unwanted uncertainty through redundancy. Yet in a critique of this model, Deleuze and Guattari (1987, 79) pose the opposite: "the redundancy of the order-word is instead primary and that information is only the minimal condition for the transmission of order-words." That is to say, language marks first and foremost a series of commands rather than communicated signs: it tells us what we *must* think through repetition or redundancy. "[It] is made not to be believed but to be obeyed, and to compel obedience" (76). For Deleuze and Guattari, "information" is thus the minimal condition to accept and relay order-words: "[o]ne must be just informed enough not to confuse 'Fire!' with 'Fore!'" (76), which makes the bare scene of contact not one of signification or exchange, but of compliance. Cultivating *intelligible* rather than *perfect* speech in deaf students describes the minimum conditions necessary to field commands and thus be "set in communication with the world." The ableist designation of "communicative" versus "non-communicative" people does not index a clear communication channel for genuine exchange, but the capacity for machinic enslavement.

In the language of Tomlinson, both telecommunications and eugenics are mobilisations of machine speed; they are rational, goal-directed projects designed to overcome resistance at biological limits. As I explained in the last chapter, SLP can quite easily produce in a stuttering body intelligible or *mechanical* speech with techniques that dramatically slow the rate of speech and remove most of its affective characteristics. In the language of information theory, mechanical speech carries less information, it is less entropic. Yet since the speed (and, as I explain in the next chapter, style) of information always figures its arrival, mechanical speech can do little more than field orders. The capacity to field and relay order-words *in the service of capital* is perhaps the minimum threshold of "inclusion" within neoliberal and communicative capitalism. Mechanical speech is easy to produce, especially in clinical conditions, but the curative imagination of SLP aims considerably higher. Mechanical speech is the first rehabilitative step towards, optimally, an effortless flow (the machinic speech I am calling fluency) that presents a stable and robust site for communicative contact, or suboptimally, a higher rate of stuttered speech in the world.

But lest we get swept into the idea that dysfluency plays a purely negative function in the pursuit of immediacy (something to be foreclosed and forgotten), it is worth asking, "What needs to slow down so we can achieve immediacy?" Here, following Sharma's (2014) work, we can recognise that privileged bodies get invested with speed (temporal value) by slowing other bodies down. Contrasting the normate business traveller who sweeps through the "temporal architecture" of the airport designed just for them, with the taxi driver who dwells outside in a time of indefinite waiting that is punctuated with bursts of speed, Sharma explains that "[s]ome populations, like taxi drivers, are in motion but are inexorably tied to a structural position within capital. They are treated as mechanical pieces of the technology that 'cradle' the valuable and producing subject, the frequent business traveler" (64). In a biopolitical economy of time, she argues, the temporal maintenance performed by populations like taxi drivers is essential insofar as they *make time* for more valuable subjects. Like capital, speed is thus vampiric. The privileges it affords to some are leached from the embodied capacities of many. Moreover, thinking with Sharma's concept of the Broken Machine, mechanical pieces of temporal architecture are *designed* to stretch and wait and wear: to cradle productive flows and absorb their excess until one's own capacity is worn beyond repair. (Recall the quip from the last chapter: "Stutterers make good workers. We don't complain!") This makes advanced capitalism a necropolitical regime insofar as it manages the maintenance, yes, but ultimately the *expiration* and *obsolescence* of its parts.

Resonant with Sharma's analysis of both temporal architecture and broken machines, Dolmage (2017, 108) argues that capitalism holds disabled populations in zones of "abeyance" or temporary and flexible suspension in order to "[pick] up or put down disabled bodies according to its needs." We witnessed this pattern already in the last chapter. Capitalism reorients the body-minds of disabled people to make their time freely available for its use, often in low-paid positions (or exploited for free), at the same time as it renders these populations front-line buffers to absorb the shocks (expressed as cutbacks and layoffs) inherent to the system. But the needs of capitalism are many. The pursuit of immediate connections manufactured on a global scale is a project that shrieks with friction and requires what Lewis Mumford (1934) calls "shock-absorbers" to decrease strain between human and machine components. Already in the nineteenth century, "the introduction of the machine was not smooth, nor were its characteristic habits of life undisputed" (311). But Mumford argues that struggles against machinic rhythms did little to slow their adoption into social life, except for the privileged few who could retreat to "private space" (shielded from speed by the temporal labour of others). Indeed, "far from stopping the machine or undermining the purely mechanical program, [such reactions] perhaps decreased the tensions that the machine produced" (312). In a similar way, I suggest that dysfluency is more than an impediment to speed; it also functions to absorb the excess of machinic contact and displace its impossible demands, and in so doing decreases the tensions produced by information machines.

In one mode, dysfluency is without question an unruly force, a dysgenic threat to mechanical speed, let alone immediacy. We can follow this idea of stuttering as "leaked energy" from the last chapter a little further by attending to the temporal dimensions of eugenics. While we often explain eugenics using spatial frameworks—topographies of bell curves and boundaries of selective immigration practices—eugenics can also be understood as the project to manage and *streamline* differential speeds of life. Francis Galton famously defined it as

> the science of improving stock, which is by no means confined to questions of judicious mating, but which, especially in the case of man, takes cognisance of all influences that tend in however remote a degree to give to the more suitable races or strains of blood a *better chance of prevailing speedily over the less suitable* than they otherwise would have had. (1883, 24–25; emphasis added)

The problematics of speed and temporality are baked into eugenics. "Less suitable" kinds of people were a danger to society precisely because they persisted through time, threatening to overtake the desirable (read: able-bodied, wealthy, white, and straight) inheritors of the future. Christina Cogdell (2004,

270) notes that for the eugenicist Charles Davenport, "defectives" were those who put the "brake on social progress," those who put a drag on machine speed.

Cogdell explains that the metaphor of a "stream" symbolising blood, inheritance, and history was highly prominent in the 1920s—the heyday of eugenics—and cites as an example the 1926 winning sermon submitted to the American Eugenic Society's annual contest by the Rev. K. S. MacArthur:

> Look at the *whirl-pools* of drift and refuse, its *eddies* of loathsome flotsam and jetsam. . . . Note its slimy scum and noisome odors. What has happened to this stream? . . . Find the impure streams of social disease, bred of vice and sin, flowing into this river of human life. See the putrefaction of criminal strains of life added to it. Note the currents and eddies of diseased mind or enfeebled intellect. (Cogdell 2004, 55–56; emphasis in original)

Whirlpools, eddies, scum, and odours result from meandering dysfluency that allows life to pool and gather in unexpected and nonproductive ways. If eugenics is the act of streamlining life in service of a transcendent value (perhaps GDP, whiteness, progress), we can imagine an intertwined ecological and counter-eugenic aspect of dysfluency that gathers life within the whirlpools of drift and refuse.

But, perhaps characteristic for a stutterer, I am getting both behind and ahead of myself. The point I want to emphasise here is that in addition to playing the role of dysgenic threat, dysfluency also functions to reduce the strain of informational bodies hurtled towards contact. I offer one example. For curious reasons, laughing about stuttering and people who stutter is often still not frowned upon.[8] Daniel Martin (2021) notes that jokes about stuttering were widespread in the nineteenth century, circulated in periodicals and, of course, everyday talk. Especially popular was the trope of two stutterers speaking to and misunderstanding each other. To consider why stuttering was and continues to be so funny, Martin (2016) turns to and interprets Henri Bergson's idea that laughter erupts when we notice "something mechanical encrusted upon the living." Martin explains in reference to stuttering:

> When artificial rhythms—stutters, hesitations, uncertainties, prats, and falls—invade the body, we recognize something in others that seems predatory in its disruption of the supposedly graceful and fluid movements of life itself. Involuntary blocks and repetitions seem funny

> to others because they make the bodies inhabiting them look inhuman or machine-like, temporarily possessed by non-human rhythms or encrusted by a broken-down thingness. (121)

In other words, we laugh at stuttering because it reminds us of those involuntary aspects of the body and life itself that jeer at the pretensions of the human subject, so graceful, smooth, and dignified. Laughter at the machine-like interaction of two stutterers trying to pair their mental content is a (yes, ultimately disablist) relief valve for the impossible demands that machines make of communicative bodies. Both discursively and materially, stuttering cushions the shocks of contact and helps to stabilise society in pursuit of immediacy. Fluent, immediate communication is cradled by broken-down things.

Controlling the (Uncontrollable) Tongue

I have suggested in this chapter that the effort to control communication through a universal turn against noise is politically charged and dangerous. I conclude with the futility of control and start from the premise that the new materialisms that matter are not passive and inert, but actants alive with their own creative force. "An actant," writes Jane Bennett, "can be human or not, most likely, a combination of both," and is that which "by virtue of its particular location in an assemblage and the fortuity of being in the right place at the right time, makes the difference, makes things happen, becomes the decisive force catalyzing an event" (2010, 9). Actants cannot exist alone, since agency is an emergent property of *relations*. Actants comingle in unexpected ways both to subtend and, at times, override human agency. This makes human agency nonexceptional; in fact, humans *only* act in federation with other actants.

Machines of control de-animate the communicative event. Bruno Latour would probably generalise this claim: modernist epistemology is profoundly de-animating because an animate world is chaotic and does not yield to representation or control. Statistical models of the world displace its *eventfulness* such that nothing can truly happen (2014, 43). Likewise, each imagined act of communication between two predefined poles and across a clear medium drains the world of agency; it affirms some actants *as* actants yet screens the force of others; it sterilises the expanse between sender and receiver in order to isolate the original intention. Dysfluency is one such actant that doesn't count. It is a material power of and over the tongue, yes, but a negative force we consider inessential or *accidental* to communication. This is why closed captions elide dysfluent repetitions or blocks: "[Stuttering] 'It wasn't me!'" The closed caption here *signals* dysfluency while transcribing the essential message and thereby contains the dysfluent event within a proxy where stuttering *represents* internal states, such as nervousness or a pathology, without any power to draw others into its becoming. The accident loses its power to derail intentions and produce spectacular crashes.

Because of such tricks that deny the multiplicity of the voice, we tend to forget that "[i]t is never an individual or even a group of individuals (intersubjectivity) who work, communicate, or produce" (Lazzarato 2014, 44). Modern communication is not simply the effect of a reduction but is *itself* a reduction machine that quells the affectivity of matter in order to trap agency in its place. Yet people who stutter know that to speak is to enter into negotiations with multiple actants over which we are never sovereign: interlocutors who fill in sentences, devices such as the SpeechEasy, power dynamics, time, stock phrases, the vestigial voices of childhood SLPs, difficult consonants, the energy of the moment, the acoustic environment, and disablist affect. Grammar can be misleading; let me stress that there is no primary voice in any assemblage of speech, no predefined intention that fights its way through other actants to arrive untarnished. The ontological force of voice *emerges* in the quality of its federation. I am here following Lisa Mazzei and Alecia Jackson's (2017, 1091) posthumanist stance that emphasises "voice as (re) configured in the intra-actions between the material and discursive, as merely one part—and perhaps the least vital component—of an agentic assemblage." The tongue is not the sovereign agent we like to imagine.

Consider that while the tongue exists as the chief index of *logos* and human sovereignty, Deleuze and Guattari insist that the mouth, tongue, and teeth do not originally belong to signification but to eating and sonority. These organs "find their primitive territoriality in food. In giving themselves over to the articulation of sounds, the mouth, tongue, and teeth deterritorialize" (1987, 19). Emissions of the body—grunts, belches, hisses—are deterritorialised noises that we have coded as articulated sound: noise captured within schemas of meaning. As Bennett (2001, 154) explains, "Language steals the mouth from eating/sonority and tries to make it pronounce/mean; language bends the sense of taste into the sense of meaning." This theft is never complete since sonority haunts signification—the phonic is never fully consumed by the phonological but remains as excess. Nevertheless, the tongue takes flight with speech. It becomes unhinged, unmoored from the material sites of enunciation, drunk on the overcoding power of signification.

Like Bennett, Hasana Sharp (2011) seeks to dethrone the sovereign human subject by attending to nonhuman actants such as chemicals, objects, and nonhuman animals. In her reading of Spinoza, Sharp asks us to appreciate the countless "bodies"—forces or affects—in the world that enable and constrain action. She admits that "speech is one of those activities that are very difficult to renaturalize" (42), and people who are fluent often imagine speech to be free from external constraint. Yet Sharp, with Spinoza, suggests that there is perhaps nothing *less* in our control. The tongue cannot be tamed. Instead of a docile instrument of the reason and will, the tongue is thrashed around by proximate forces in the environment, mostly outside the conscious register. Spinoza writes that

> human affairs, of course, would be conducted far more happily if it were equally in man's power to be silent and to speak. But experience teaches all too plainly that men have *nothing less* in their power than their tongues, and can do nothing less than moderate their appetites. (1994; cited in Sharp 47)

As a case study we might consider the white male philosopher [*homo rationalist*] perched in his habitat, the colloquium, tongue vibrating, simply unable to contain itself. "What Spinoza underscores is that the affects exciting tongues are as powerful as an alcoholic's urge for whiskey or an infant's yearning for milk. They can hardly be resisted" (Sharp 48). We shame dysfluent tongues for their indocility yet conveniently forget that fluent tongues are not *ruled* by self-transparent intentions but *excited* by affective assemblages. The tongue is habituated within a common sense to reproduce dominant opinions and ways of speaking. In short, "we imagine ourselves to cause our words, when we have little if any understanding—let alone mastery—of the vast multiplicity of causes that incite our speech" (47). This warning should provoke pause, especially within a so-called information society so sure of its fluency.

How then can the unmasterable tongue be governed? Spinoza famously defends free speech, but as Sharp notes, this is because human speech is *not* free—because the tongue is irrepressible. "Since what we say does not flow from mental decrees over which we have independent control," she explains, "it is futile and self-undermining for a government to legislate the appropriateness of speech acts, or spoken passions" (52). However, while it might be futile for a sovereign power (which relates to its subjects as an exteriority) to legislate verbal passions in attempts to plug the mouth, the abstract machines of the control society bypass this problem. Control societies *manu-*

facture proximate bodies to send information running within networks of global telecommunications captured by capital. Recall that Deleuze (1990, 137) warns of those "forces making us say things when we've nothing much to say," while Sharp reminds us, from the other side, of the very irrepressibility of the tongue. The inhuman forces of control societies expertly exploit the tongue. For Sharp, the unruliness of the tongue offers an invitation to become aware of *and account for* the multiple forces that enable and constrain action within the concreteness of the event. This is a generative way to listen, and I suggest that we expand this awareness to include the inhuman machines at work that incite endless communication.

Control societies work directly on material flows to amplify and speed the circulation of information. Why legislate the tongue when its powers can be captured and redirected into networks of profit and control? Phillipe Breton (2011) likens the information age to a deluge that brings to the surface hidden sediment and sweeps away all impediment to circulation. He writes: "The actual annihilation of the 'non-visible,' deemed opaque, cannot help but be an attack on barriers, frontiers, on all separations which impede the flow of information, the 'generalized interconnection' and the final transparency of the world" (63). The war against noise leaves its marks on the body. People who do not communicate verbally or are literally too ashamed of their voice to leave the house or make a call, for example, represent challenges to the project of transparency; they are neo-eugenic frontiers to annihilate.

We can frame the challenge more tightly: the demand to communicate without cessation (to poise tongues always for activation) must ultimately, I argue, be read alongside the neoliberal reduction of all things to the logic and form of capital. Wendy Brown (2015) argues that neoliberalism works to detach speech from the source of enunciation to make it acquire the features of and operate like capital itself. As an example, we might consider with Brown the 2012 US Supreme Court ruling in *Citizens United v. FEC*. This landmark case ruled that spending money was a form of disseminating speech such that the government could not restrict corporations from contributing money to political campaigns. Brown suggests that this ruling equates speech with capital in two ways: "Speech is *like* capital in its natural, irrepressible, dynamic, and creative nature." Like capital, speech is not simply a general equivalent that represents reality but a creative force that gives it shape. At the same time, "speech operates *as* capital to enhance the positioning of its bearer in . . . the 'political marketplace'" (162). The function of speech becomes, like capital, to appreciate value and advance its bearer's interest. Neoliberalism holds the circulation of speech, like capital, to be an axiomatic good such that *any* restriction of information—from the State or disabled body—is a harm, while any attempt to redistribute power and produce substantive rather than formal equality in the "political marketplace" is "simply to make a Keynesian moral and technical error" (162). To control the circulation of speech, in a negative sense, is to deny its nature. But to make speech free, we must subject it to (positive) control. This is the paradox: control captures communication to set it free; it *forces* communication to be free on its austere terms of service. Austerity introduces a feedback loop—a de-livened world de-livens our sensitivity to other bodies, which in turn de-livens the world.

One way beyond this feedback loop is to retune ourselves to the affectivity of matter. If control is a failed dream, let us find strategies that focus rather than deny the agency of bodies. In closing, let me offer and appraise two.

First, we might consider Virilio's (1997) idea that information societies need, in addition to the "freedom of expression," a robust account of "freedom of perception." He reasons that since information pollution is now so widespread, it would surely "[b]e appropriate to entertain a kind of *right to blindness*, just as there is already a right to relative deafness or, at least, to a lowering of the noise level in shared space, public places" (96; emphasis in original). Although most likely unintended, this is an interesting claim given the history of the ugly laws and the public's right *from* disability. The freedom to contest our exposure to information intrigues me, and I agree in a rough sense that less general noise can facilitate modes of being-with. The problem is that Virilio invokes disability as a limit to perception and thus limits his own critique. Disability is a trope that represents a right to *a lower intensity of the same* rather than a right to genuine difference.

Construed as such, freedom of sight or sound perception might allow us to perceive and relate in different ways, but might just as easily insulate us from disability and becoming-other.

To employ a distinction made by Mack Hagood (2019, 233), freedom of perception tends towards "hearing what we want," instead of "wanting what we hear." As someone who regularly uses noise-cancelling headphones to work, I understand the desire for selective hearing. But I have also been the noise: the actant cancelled by headphones on public transit. Without addressing the ultimately counter-eugenic question of desire—that is, what and how we *want* to hear—the "right from perception" (a right, ostensibly, *for* disability) could in theory be satisfied by curative technologies such as either noise-cancelling headphones or the SpeechJammer. Both deafness and dysfluency are useful tools of control when torn from their terrestrial relations. Deafness on demand; dysfluency on demand. Stuck in the mode of closed listening, of "hearing what we want," the right to disability is thus really the right to its annihilation and not much else: the right to deafness is the right to cancel ugly voices; the right to dysfluency is the right to silence.

Instead of "hearing what we want," Hagood invites us to consider the second, more generative strategy in the terms of what Kate Lacey (2013) calls "adventurous hearing." This is to be open to "voices that are unfamiliar or uneasy on the ear" (197). Like freedom from perception, this practice is tuned to the receptiveness of bodies and recognises that dysfluency can stir uncomfortable affect. The difference is that adventurous listening is mobilised by what I would call a counter-eugenic impulse. It resists the temptation to recoil from the embodied event of dysfluency and invites a mutual becoming. This practice draws on what Franco Berardi (2011) calls the faculty of "sensibility," which he contrasts with that of "sensitivity." Sensitivity, Berardi explains, is "the ability of the human senses to process information," while sensibility describes "the power to interpret a continuum of non-discrete elements, nonverbal signs, and the flows of empathy" (22). The faculty of sensitivity *requires* a deadened world with clear guardrails to speed the flow of information between its nodes. Over time, discouraging sensibility and inhabiting milieus of connection (where sensibility is damaging and shunned as a child of entropy) dulls the faculty. This is one cost of maintaining "competitive efficiency" in a deterritorialised field of information.

Sensibility is inefficient and thus, Berardi argues, is *inhibited* within connective milieus. Safe practices of listening that recode boundaries are essential to connection since "[e]ach element remains distinct and interacts only functionally" (39). Sensibility, on the other hand, implies that entities conjoin and *become something other* through intra-action. This is the practice of adventurous hearing, one that engages rather than flattens dysfluency. The sensible faculty is intrinsic to many crip modes of communication. In the spirit of inviting coalition, we might start to imagine the wide range of crips who speak dysfluently: deaf speech, cerebral palsy speech, lisping, autistics communicating through pictures, AAC, echolalia, and hand flapping, elders forgetting their words or mumbling, mad digressions, vocal tics . . . again, this is less a list (certainly not exhaustive!) and more an invitation to listen across identitarian boundaries.

Although we might push back against the demand for communication and signification, to enter into nonverbal communication nevertheless requires imagination and courage. Machines that inhibit sensibility and render ambiguity and slowness not only useless but *dangerous* to "communication" change the material conditions of possibility of being-together and intra-action. In a more specific sense, they restrict how dysfluency can connect and what it can connect with. We are all decontextualised voices that connect smoothly and compete "equally" within fields of scarce attention.

But there is no code that can standardise this type of listening, since it is by definition an openness to ambiguity, to uncertainty, and especially to the boundaries of *bad* uncertainty. Listening in this mode, we might begin to hear differently and thus hear difference itself. We might, with Carol Padden (2015, 45), hear that the disabled body "does not merely attempt to communicate, but by [its] realignment of [itself] with material and communicative resources, [it compels] new forms of engagement and interaction." No longer accidental, no longer a limit to perception, nonuniversal embodiments that demand something of us within the ambiguous event of communication can, quite literally, re-matter what matters.

The obstacles to any experimentation are those clerics of information who attend to the machines of compulsory fluency and never stop asking, "Yes, but in the end, wouldn't you rather be more like me?" (McRuer 2006, 382). Why would anyone *desire* noise or the breakdown of communication? But perhaps the question we should be asking is this: Who does fluency benefit? What does it achieve? In his Deleuzian reading of information, Kane Faucher (2013, 231) rightly notes that "Practically speaking, when dealing with technology, it is perhaps a favourable desire to reduce noise and stave off entropy." I hate it as much as anyone when calls drop and Zoom conversations are delayed or fuzzy. But a shift occurs when we insist on machinic norms as a *normative social category*. Faucher continues:

> Again, the genealogical question arises here in discerning *for whom* is such a desire worthy? The answer is clearly *for us*, yet it is one thing to construct machines that can reduce noise and ensure some degree of reliable function, and quite another to map this onto life in its entirety, reterritorializing life according to the same demands we apply to our technological instruments. (231; emphasis in original)

The premise here is that the free flow of information will benefit society as a whole—the neoliberal rising tide that (one day TBD!) will smooth over inequality. But this "for us" can never be taken for granted; it is a category of differential inclusion within networks of info-capital.

Deleuze rejects the conceptual ecologies of both "information" and "communication" precisely because these regimes posit entropy as enemy rather than a condition of the possibility of life. Risk management contains becoming. The first and essential act of communicative contact is to reduce the uncertainty of an event to a "set of more or less probable states and alternatives as constrained by the interplay between a channel and a code" (Terranova 2004, 24). These discourses operationalise possible connections and eliminate chance. With Nietzsche, Deleuze rather desires the positive affirmation of chance and difference. He suggests a "counter-actualization," or the re-working of the event to introduce a difference within repetition and release the virtual potentials of an assemblage. Counter-actualisation is a practice closely related to what Guattari terms an existential affirmation, which I take up in the conclusion. I will suggest that we imagine dysfluency as a form of parrhesia—courageous or honest or *risky* speech that, among other things, creates a territory. What might escape in a dysfluent event that is not immediately operationalised as channel/code, signal and noise? What might we become? How might we relate differently? Here we might imagine the body as an experiment, a risk *without guarantee of return.*

Three

Becoming Talking Heads

On television, you are always in danger of being trapped in the dominant meanings and subjectivations, no matter what you say or do. You speak, but you run the risk of saying nothing of what really matters to you.
—Lazzarato

So far, we have examined two *dispositifs* that emerged from liberal commitments and frameworks to regulate the communicative body: speech-language pathology and communication sciences. While these regimes have always flirted, it is now time to recognize that under neoliberalism they have joined to produce something new: what I call an "info-therapeutic" regime populated by, officially, talking heads. Info-therapeusis calibrates and mobilizes SLP to serve the specific demands of information machines. As a popular handbook for broadcasting states: "*The first rule of the TV screen, radio airtime, and print advertising is that nothing is there by accident*" (Eastman 2006, 128; emphasis in original). I suggested earlier in this book that the talking head is a clearing. Because nothing can be by accident, the good talking head must accordingly be *made* by high priests of information—trained to fit within frames, to look good, to be fully controlled, and to hold attention within specific parameters. Virilio (1999), for example, contends that Bill Clinton had to be coached by experts to appeal to the screen: his true addressee. "Obeying strict television rules, he had to be able to say everything on a particular theme in less than ninety seconds—before going on to say nothing at all about it after he was elected" (75). What is the talking head? A product and instrument of info-therapeusis; a spigot of cheap talk.

The first section of this chapter characterises the talking head and locates its production in an info-therapeutic regime. The second section turns to examine the *function* of the talking head, where I argue that the talking head (1) passes along "order-words" and (2) smooths relations. But taken as a whole, I suggest that talking heads perform a unique priestly function. The generic role of a priest is to serve as an intermediary between the populace and the divine and/or the elite class. The priest is privy to what happens beyond the veil of power and thus speaks *for* and attends *to* the divine (and/or elite class) in their rites and service for the community. While I have referred throughout this book to both SLPs and media technocrats as priests of the information age, this is not the entire story. These are the *high* priests over the bodies of information, yes, but we are *all* priests of a different sort.

The initial waves of information theory and the early years of the Web expressed profound optimism about the potential of free-flowing information to level hierarchical forms of power, whether they be state or religious. In this regard, the sixteenth- and twentieth-century revolutions in information are much alike: both cybernetics and the Protestant Reformation were revolutions of the priestly class. Luther, and those who followed, sought to abolish the elite class of Roman Catholic priests who alone could read the Bible and access truth. The "universal priesthood of all believers" remains a central tenet of Protestantism and was a democratising force made possible in part by the printing press, in a way resembling how access to the internet affords (in theory) a democratisation of knowledge and has produced its own new priestly class. While some claim this birthright more zealously than others, we are today all born into a universal priesthood of information that extends not merely the right but the *duty* to connect and circulate information. I turn in the later part of the chapter to examine the normative aspects of this priesthood of talking heads, for while it is an important countereugenic trend, the increased access to information has also introduced grave dangers. But by way of introduction, consider one conceit of this birthright: its universality.

Vignette 9: Connectivity as Human Right

In 2010, Mark Zuckerberg underscored the popular adage—"if it's free, you are the product"—by publishing a manifesto called "Is Connectivity a Human Right?" The Facebook CEO noted that only 1/3 of the world's population has internet access and framed his corporate vision to close this digital divide as an issue of human rights. Yet while cloaked in human-rights discourse, Zuckerberg had nothing to say about equity, connectivity, the human subject of rights, or even rights themselves. The question—is connectivity a human right?—was a pre-made question that came with a pre-made answer in order to greenlight Facebook's corporate vision to bring more of the world's population into its digital economy. "The internet," he writes, "not only connects us to our friends, families and communities, but it is also"—now addressing not the talking heads, but his shareholders in their own language—"the foundation of the global knowledge economy" (2).

Vignette 10: Disturbing Disconnections

Ability Access is the UK's largest disability Facebook page. In early 2019, this community posted an image of Vicky Balch, a white woman, proudly displaying her disabled body. In the picture, Balch is unclothed, though the image is not explicit; her amputated right leg is clearly visible. While this image was empowering for Balch and others, the algorithms of Facebook flagged the image and then blocked the group. Seeking resolution, Simon Sansome, the creator of Ability Access, contacted Facebook's marketing team, and this dialogue ensued:

> FB: [. . .] Anything that could be disturbing . . . is-is-is-um, is-is not allowed by Facebook, on-on by the algorithm.
> SS: Well, dis-disability is not disturbing; disability is a fact of life.
> FB: Well even, *you, you will have to understand it* in a way like, um, some people find it, find it disturbing to see pictures of disabled people, for example. *You will have to think about it like that.* Even for me personally it wouldn't be disturbing, but for many other people. . . . It is how the algorithm picks it out [. . . .] (Sansome 2019; transcription and emphasis mine)

The marketing team, insisting they could not help, instructed Ability Access to review the policy and send their complaint to technical support. A "Facebook spokesperson" later offered a profuse apology for the first statement and scrambled to the high ground that the post was rejected simply for "depicting adult content"—making sure we know that Facebook takes pride in Ability Access for using their platform to "reach people."

• • •

Who belongs to this priesthood of connection? Or better: who belongs to which stream of the priesthood? The first vignette paints from a Zuck's-eye view a utopia of connection; the second is the lived and more sober reality for bodies that do not connect in predictable ways. Let me be clear: this water is murky. Social media have offered avenues for people historically marginalised from both social life and the cultural imagination to gain visibility and increase their power to act. Precisely because social media platforms seem to snub their noses at overproduction—the idea cited above that "nothing is there by accident"—disabled and nonnormatively bodied peoples have often engaged social media as technologies of empowerment.

The point of friction I want to draw our attention to is that insofar as these technologies are necessarily embedded in dynamics of social power, transgressive or "disturbing" bodies struggle at once against disablism and to gain visibility. This issue is not restricted to one platform. TikTok recently admitted that its algorithms had been concealing video content from disabled, fat, and queer talking heads who, they assert, are "vulnerable to cyberbullying" (Botella 2019). We could, of course, question the PR spin, much like we could spend time unpacking the disablist narratives that mealy-mouthed corporate talk circulates. But I here want to make a different point: the right to full membership in the universal priesthood of information that Zuckerberg touts rests on a conceit.

Both the Protestant and cybernetic revolutions were attempts to seize their epistemic means of production—to access information (the Bible or internet) unprocessed by religious or state machinations. Both sought shared ownership over the procedures of meaning-making and world-building—access to information, to codes, that do not simply represent but *shape* the world. I will leave the Protestant success or failure aside; for the cybernetic revolution, the failure to seize the algorithmic means of production has become obvious. Or rather, the neoliberal capture is nearly complete. Zuckerberg feigns a democratisation of information when he insists that a knowledge economy is not zero sum. "If you know something, that doesn't stop me from knowing it too. In fact, the more things we all know, the better ideas, products and service we can all offer and the better all of our lives will be" (2010, 2). Shut the Zuck up. I will take his sentiment seriously when Facebook shares its own data freely. Info-capitalism is predicated on the constant enclosure of source code and ideas, which requires access to a semiotic common to exploit. These, then, are the two strata of informational priesthood: first, the high priests who have access to secret knowledge (e.g., market research, source code, algorithms) and thus control the epistemic means of production; second, a universal rank of demi-priests whose primary function is to attend to the needs of information machines. The conceit is that there exists only one priesthood and, moreover, that the machine serves *us*.

But notice how the first spokesperson for Facebook that Ability Access contacted defers to the objective authority of the machines, the algorithms, with a tone that approaches reverence. "Anything that could be disturbing . . . is-is-is-um, is-is not allowed by Facebook, on-on by the algorithm." The high priesthood answers to the algorithms. Their job is to interpret the machines' desires and execute them as orders, which is evident in the spokesperson's repeated use of the imperative to which they too are bound: "*you will have to think about it like that.*" To enter the priesthood of info-therapeusis is to adopt the perspective (the desires and protocols) of the machines. The conditional nature of the imperative is implied: you, a talking head, will have to think like the machines . . . or else you will be disconnected, dissembled, and thrown into the pile of broken machines. McRuer (2006, 8) insists that within industrial capitalist systems, one is "free to sell one's labor but not free to do anything else," which effectively means being "free to have an able body but not particularly free to have anything else." Within a *post*-industrial system, it might be that we are free to "connect" in normative ways—free to be a talking head—but not free to do much else. As I will argue in the conclusion of this chapter, we are free to access and circulate information in the mode of consumption, but not to ask about or transform its conditions.

Info-therapeusis, then, is the collision of two neoliberal forces: individualising therapeutic practices and de-individualising processes of machinic enslavement. Therapeusis is a "velvet cage" (McFalls and Pandolfi 2014, 170) since it deploys self-disciplinary mechanisms such as self-care and self-maintenance. Despite its soft touch, therapeusis still reinscribes dominant norms on bodies and minds, making them compliant to instrumental control in the name of an impersonal well-being and happiness. Therapeusis frames representation as empowering, but, thinking like the machine, the self-maintenance that especially marginalised individuals perform on themselves to become talking heads has nothing to do with personal expression or empowerment. The "technologics" of power (Sharma 2020, 172) bend therapeusis to their own designs. Becoming a serviceable talking head is to think, speak, and listen like the machine and thus be *capable* of offering it service.

Moten and Harney (2013) argue that from a critical race perspective, capitalism has always possessed various ways to make bodies work, and that the subject is a recent invention restricted to a small subset of *Homo sapiens*. The Atlantic slave trade, the plantation—*these* are the models of capitalist appropriation without the subject. What they term "logistics" references the "ambition to connect bodies, objects, affects, information, without subjects, without the formality of subjects" (92). One goal of logistics is to remove the human agent from the equation of governance and exploitation. The subject is too clumsy for control. It moves with too much pomp—demanding formal recognition and rights. It is thus, Moten and Harney write, that "[l]ogistical populations will be created to do without thinking, to feel without emotion, to move without friction, to adapt without question, to translate without pause, to connect without interruption, or they will be dismantled and disabled as bodies in the same way they are assembled" (91). The talking head is a product of info-therapeusis, an entity of logistical populations that is hollow, designed not to understand or judge but to connect, translate, and circulate.

This chapter careens toward a spectacular accident: building universal access to information highways is a crucial strategy from the perspective of disability justice, but at the same time, removing barriers to online participation has arguably incubated a priesthood of talking heads that, as Deleuze would say, plague the world with pointless statements thoroughly unconnected from their problematics. But to question *if* the priesthood *should* be universal introduces hierarchies infused with a eugenic logic (e.g., are there "kinds" of people who shouldn't get to participate in public discourse?) that sit at odds with critical disability studies. This is the collision towards which we speed and that we must untangle. I thus conclude by reflecting on access and friction in the context of Deleuze and Guattari's (1987, 500) warning to "[n]ever believe that a smooth space will suffice to save us."

Features of the Talking Head

I use "talking head" in a fairly loose sense to highlight links between practices and concepts that might otherwise go unnoticed. The talking head, in the most general sense, is a machine that forms connections with other semiotic components. It *relays* information to form connections and is, as such, fluent in multiple mediums. Audio and audiovisual are the most familiar—the disembodied voice of the radio newscaster that reads scripts, the gridwork of pundits cut at the shoulders who argue on cable news—but, although important differences exist, we might also consider the hyper-poster on Facebook or Twitter, always wedged in the thick of the flow, poised for their "hot take" on every circumstance. Control incites communication wherever and whenever possible, such that talking heads work mixed semiotics; they exercise, not the ability to wax poetic, but the flexible capacity to move between and intervene in these flows, mobilising the power of networks.

Dysfluent people know from experience as faulty talking heads that bodies are not functional wholes but dissembled organs. We exist as deterritorialised bodies of communication (a wobbly federation of tongues, hands, faces, lungs) that must somehow form a talking head that can compete for attention—*to not be noise*—in an informational field devoid of context. We are an awkward assemblage of organs that know the strict limits of (in)human attention. This is true both phenomenologically and machinically. Drew Leder (1990, 122) explains that phenomenologically, "the minimal materiality of linguistic signs demands only a minimal though intricate use of the body." However, when something goes "wrong"—like when one blocks hard on a word mid-conversation—the organs of the body *dys*-appear or rush to the forefront to become hyper-present. The face scrunches, the lungs tighten, and the body can convulse as it takes on a more active role in language. The stutterer experiences their body as an assemblage of organs only partially under control. And, if "the body itself is not a point but an organized field in which certain organs and abilities come to prominence while others recede" (24), then in addition to the phenomenological field we can also imagine a global, machinic field of communicative organs where there is no whole or centre but simply connections.

There is no essence of a machine—only operations of which it is capable—such that offering a list of the characteristics of talking heads seems quite pointless. But there is, nevertheless, a cluster of common attributes of good talking heads. If the "proper speech" of the nineteenth century was produced by technologies of elocution that referenced humanist norms and striated class, race, gender, and ability, then what we might call "machinic speech" is that indexed to the pragmatic or *operating* norms that make machines run smoothly. Machinic speech serves a different function than proper speech. It does not distinguish, but smooths; it effaces bodies into circulation. In the last chapter I mapped the noise-free channel as a neutral medium that facilitates the "free" exchange of information. But we can now ask a different question: what does this clean relation *do* or *enable to be done*?

First, more than a medium for exchange, the noise-free channel is **executable**: it converts meaning to action. Machinic speech is a thoroughly pragmatic language that intervenes in the machinic assemblage of bodies. Voice-operated machines like Google Home or Amazon Echo use "human" voices to trigger a complex series of protocols bundled into a female human persona that can perform a multitude of tasks. Voiced words are simply inputs: if . . . then. What a sign means (or could mean) is less important than its function—what operations it can perform.

Second, picking up a theme from the last chapter, the machinic tongue is **interoperable**. This refers to the capacity of systems to interface and exchange information. "In order to connect, segments must be compatible and open to interfacing and interoperability" (Berardi 2011, 39–40). The good talking head endlessly circulates and translates in order to produce new relations and fields of attention, and to do so must conform itself to homogenising codes. It is by flattening the indeterminacy of voices and patterns of communication—as well as imposing neurotypical cues and body languages—that otherwise heterogeneous surfaces and processes are made connectible.

Third, revisiting another theme, machinic speech is **fast**. The clarity or iterability of a message does not matter if it arrives too slowly. Falling behind a conversation, I often feel my dysfluent speech to arrive late and thus never truly arrive at all. Remi Yergeau (2018, 60) explains that autistic people are stamped with *kakoethos* or a "marked and stigmatic presence." Those with "kakoethical character," they write, "cannot escape their demi-rhetorical suspension, even if their rhetorical impairments are mere matters of degree, or mildness. Kakoethos forever impedes rhetorical arrival" (60). The dysfluent rhetor is similar in this regard. The stigma attached to my body does more than reduce the time I may occupy, it slows the arrival of the message enough that it never really arrives.

The problem of arrival intensifies when bodies are subject to the inhuman speeds of immediacy. Virilio (1999, 141) insists that "slowed-up information [is] no longer even worthy of that name, but mere background noise." For example, to have their journalism *count* as news in a hypersaturated world of twenty-four-hour coverage, talking heads must not only keep pace with global events, but with their competitors. An anxious and competitive fear of becoming noise thus fuels the rush towards immediacy, the rush *of* immediacy. Speed is the true message, since "digital messages and images matter less than their instantaneous delivery; the 'shock effect' always wins out over the consideration of the informational content" (141). Nevertheless, the manufacture of affective shock produces diminishing returns, and this, Mumford (1934, 316) argues, is one reason cultural shock-absorbers are essential for the machines: "the shock-absorber prepares one for a fresh shock"; it resets the potential for contact.

Emerging from the problem of maintaining contact (at speed and with shock effect), the machinic tongue must have **style**. Info-therapeutics work to machine the talking head to fit its needs. Having functionally smooth speech—articulate, pragmatic, interoperable, and accelerable—is thus a necessary but not sufficient condition for a good talking head. Style attracts attention, it whets appetites, such that the machines that incite communication *encourage* a plurality of unique and even nonnormative talking heads in order to maximise market share of collective attention—if they can follow the dictates of info-therapeusis.

The good talking head, then, is an assemblage of organs primed to communicate, to compete to connect and make contact, in psychosocial *economies of attention*. While the office, school, or factory requires sustained attention (recall from chapter 1 that these disciplinary regimes sprung many leaks), information societies fragment attention into ever smaller pieces to maximise both semiotic exposure and the speed of circulation. What Jeffrey Scheuer (2001, 8) terms the "Sound Bite Society" is one "flooded with images and slogans, bits of information and abbreviated or symbolic messages—a culture of instant but shallow communication." Scheuer describes the field of deterritorialised language and bodies, of part-signs and split attention. It is the short yet memorable slogans that cut through the noise to establish contact. Within this busy yet sterile ecology of attention, one must, the priests all say, join the conversation as a talking head to exercise power. *Make your voice heard.* As I argued in the last chapter, language steals the mouth to signify rather than eat. The talking head continues this process, ripping the organs of signification from the body and tethering them to the protocols of information machines.[1]

The talking head uproots from the earth to become a vehicle, a terminal, of information. This is made possible when cybernetics disconnects hearing, seeing, and speaking from singular, embodied, sources in order to treat them as isolated and thus automatable functions. Speaking and listening both become *predictive* rather than *responsive*. The way that algorithms predict (and thus standardise, making automatic) input in the form of autotype mirrors how fluent people "finish" dysfluent sentences, predicting and interjecting based on standardising protocols rather than making space for something new to emerge. In becoming-automatic, speaking and hearing reduce to technical problems of signals and stimuli, which in turn become pulsating inputs and outputs in global systems of communication. "The functions, organs, and strengths of man are connected with certain functions, organs and strengths of the technical machine and together they constitute an arrangement" (Lazzarato 2006). Decoded or "freed up" in the form of information, the tongue (along with other organs) can thus enter new assemblages that remap the body—its powers and possibilities primed to circulate information and affect.[2]

But despite these transformations to the body, I want to be careful not to posit a natural and somehow unprocessed mode of perception now encrusted with information technologies. William Connolly (2002, 27) explains that ordinary perceptions are always geared towards the range of possible action in one's world, such that perceptions *necessarily* arrive to us pre-processed by very speedy, preconscious functions of the body/brain that have already filtered out irrelevant sensory data and patterned what remains. Attention to the differential speeds within (what Connolly calls) the body/brain/culture network wards off the idea that everyday perception is less processed and thus (somehow) more objective than its machinic counterpart. Connolly makes explicit the connection between ordinary perception and watching TV: "In both TV-mediated settings and action-orientated situations, a host of sensory material must be reduced and processed by a technocultural apparatus to render perception possible" (24). While this connection is for Connolly an invitation to explore the process of perception through film, he finds television a less promising avenue:

> Part of the reason is that its news programs and talk shows are dominated by talking heads who purport to report things as they are, even as they sometimes expose "bias" in other shows or politicians. The cumulative result of this combination is that simple objectivity is set up as the gold standard of perception, while critics accuse each other of failing to live up to it. This game of mutual recrimination set against a simple standard of objectivity, in turn, fosters the public cynicism that many TV talking heads purport to resist. (24–5)

Becoming a vehicle for "simple objectivity" that obscures the very conditions of perception is an adaptive advantage for talking heads scrambling for capital in a sound-bite society. Especially for elite (authorised) talking heads, style correlates with trustworthiness and "truthiness." According to Nimmo and Combs (1992, 25), the single qualification for membership in the priesthood of punditry is acceptance as an acolyte, which "hinges chiefly on the capacity of the new Brahman members to exhibit (as in exhibitionist) mastery of the style, language, and confidence of the priesthood." Mastering info-therapeutic norms is here a rite of initiation into a priesthood charged with power to report the world as it is. But, thinking with Connolly, the public—the *universal* priesthood—is already in on the game and thus recognises simple objectivity for the scam it is. The smooth talker poisons the soil of truth-telling and sows the ground for both trolls and yet more (but now authentic!) talking heads.

The Priestly Functions of Talking Heads

The partition between the characteristics and functions of the talking head is thin, and I have already tracked muddy feet all over the threshold. Nevertheless, with some general features sketched in, we can put these ideas to work and turn to the more interesting question: What does the talking head do? Or, *what are its priestly functions?* I pick out two related functions of the universal priesthood: passing order words and smoothing. But first, it is important to examine the priesthood itself, including its hierarchy of high and low priests. For while on paper the universal priesthood blasts apart hierarchies by claiming that everyone can "join the conversation," important divisions of power remain that the high priesthood of info-therapeusis works hard to obscure.

Allow me to introduce a second model of communication to help make my point. Much of the argument in this book has been tuned to what James Carey (2009) calls the "transmission model." But alongside this dominant model of communication persists what Carey calls the "ritual view" of communication. He explains: "if the archetypal case of communication under a transmission view is the extension of messages across geography for the purpose of control, the archetypal case under a ritual view is the sacred ceremony that draws persons together in fellowship and commonality" (15). The church, rather than the telegraph office; the chant rather than the message. In the mode of ritual, communication is the shared act of constructing, maintaining, and celebrating common worlds (Lipardi 2014, 12). In this regard, the priestly function of the talking head is more than relaying information in the form of sound bites; through repetition of phrases (mantras, prayers, liturgies), the talking head establishes and sustains a shared, yet very particular, world. Carey explains that in the mode of ritual, "news is not information but drama. It does not describe the world but portrays an arena of dramatic forces and action; it exists solely in historical time; and it invites our participation on the basis of our assuming, often vicariously, social roles within it" (17). One notable danger of the priesthood of talking heads is their conflation of "neutral" transmission and their participation in the arena of dramatic forces. A priesthood busy shepherding their "contending forces in the world" (16) while also reifying a mode of speaking and listening unmoored from a common world is an erosive force in social and mental ecologies.

It is typical for priesthoods to form hierarchies that correspond to their multiple social and religious functions. Although the *idea* of a universal priesthood drove the Protestant revolution, it nevertheless produced its own high priests, such as Luther and Calvin. An essential difference is this: the universal priesthood could now access the holy text, but this was "read-only access." High priests, on the other hand, had permission to read, write, and execute (e.g., Luther questioned both the interpretation and the very canon of the Bible). High priests access, interpret, and at times edit holy texts. They have access to the social elite and the divine itself. Their words, in the form of special rites and precepts, are charged with power. Lesser priests, on the other hand, service gods in the mundane ways that keep the machine running: lighting candles, reciting prayers, offering care, hearing confession, circulating holy words. These priests are *marked* with the authority of the divine but only channel its power in superficial ways. Thus, despite the fact that universal priesthoods are meant to level epistemic playing fields, the ostensible levelling of the priesthood actually papers over declensions of power.

We can trace a similar division of priestly labour in the twenty-first century, noting that while the entire priesthood engages in the labour of world-building with communication machines, there is a division of labour (and access to information) between the high priests of info-therapeusis and the lower, universal class of talking heads. Philippe Breton (2011, 39) explains that the information society "has left the circle of specialists who gave it birth and now reaches a vast public. The cult of information has been realized and popularized *via* the cult of the Internet." Communication machines must be regularly maintained, repaired, optimised, and accelerated. Some aspects of this service are handled by specialists, the high priests, who can interpret the language of the machine, while mundane service they delegate to the talking heads. What is this routine service? These machines are insatiable and must be fed a steady influx of data (clicks, content, and geo-tagged posts) and be stroked to excitation (likes, comments, and shares) to keep everything in flow. The act of servicing an infinite debt of data to the communicative machine is the primary duty of the talking heads, one they exercise not in a haze of incense but with drugs of other kinds. The controlled drip of serotonin and dopamine, yes, but also the false taste of power (that of immediacy) which stirs this priesthood into the religious fervour of endless contact and chatter. Through their service, heads are torn from their own sites of enunciation and absorbed as talking organs, component parts, into the operation of the machine.

These differences in priestly duties emerge not from intrinsic individual characteristics, but from segregated streams of capital, knowledge, and semiotics. By restricting talking heads to an "impotent" flow of signs (Deleuze and Guattari 1983, 228), the high priests of info-therapeusis can safely universalise the lower priesthood—everyone join the conversation!—and grant themselves unfettered access to an exploitable semiotic common and a surplus of replaceable parts. It is such that the universality of the cybernetic revolution is characterised by differential inclusion. The vital question is not

Table 1

Flows Easily Accessed by High Priests	**Flows Easily Accessed by Low Priests**
Capital-Money	Payment-Money
Investment-Knowledge	Payment-Knowledge
Asignifying Signs	Signifying Signs
Power-Speech	Payment-Speech

"*Are* you a talking head?" but "*How good* a talking head are you?" Whether we like it or not, we all belong to this priesthood. This is true even for those on the other side of the digital divide, for as Zuckerberg makes clear in the opening vignette, those without internet access or info-therapeutic literacy are talking-heads-in-waiting. And, moreover, similar to how the therapeutic influence of SLP radiates across an entire population, so info-therapeusis habituates talking heads to perform (sound bites) for the screen whether it is on or off.

It is true that talking heads regularly break and get dissembled for their parts. What to do with a broken machine no longer connected to flows is a thoroughly political question. But despite the glitches and breakdowns, our collective faith in connectivity remains quite unshakeable. This faith is yet another product of our priestly duties. The seeming universality of information flow can, if one squints, make democracy itself feel nearly complete, as if, under the banner of communicative inclusion and participation, economic and social justice is just a few more conversations away. Discussion or dialogue becomes a technocratic fix—an instance of neoliberalism's "technohubris" (Homer-Dixon 2000, 247)—which makes it important to attend to the stratifications of priestly power and offer a sober assessment of the limits of our priestly power as talking heads. Toward this end, I sketch a set of contrasts within the "universal" priesthood.

We can first notice that the two priesthoods draw from different forms of money: capital and exchange, distinguished only by their function. Capital-money flows in the circuit of M-C-M (Money-Commodity-Money) as an *investment* in labour and society. It is capital-money that holds power to create and direct the future: understood in its purest and most speculative form as "M-M" ("Money-Money") where it drops commodity production to draw a return on *any* type of flow. The bio and tech industries are prime frontiers for speculative capital. Exchange-money, on the other hand, is an impotent sign of *payment* (of both commodities and debt). Exchange-money simply facilitates this contract; we sell commodities (mainly our own labour, packets of time, and data) to get money to buy other commodities—Commodity-Money-Commodity. As a form of general equivalence, it has no power to influence the future.[3]

Second, Jean-François Lyotard (1984) accents the heterogeneity of money in his critique of knowledge and suggests that learning circulates similarly to money: in the form of both "payment knowledge" and "investment knowledge." We can imagine that some channels of knowledge "would be reserved for the 'decision makers,' while the others would be used to repay each person's perpetual debt with respect to the social bond" (6). We have, on the one hand, the specialist scientific, managerial, and technocratic knowledges that reproduce asymmetry. This stream of knowledge taps into speculative capital and is distinctly productive, although it functions primarily to increase worker efficiency and overall optimise the performance of systems. Payment knowledge, on the other hand, simply services our infinite debt to the social bond. Like exchange money, payment knowledge functions as a simple mediation between equivalents—the equal liberal human subject of language. Payment knowledge is used to carry out orders and reproduce the material conditions of life/society. James Marshall (1999, 309) takes Lyotard to mean that education is "no longer concerned with the pursuit of ideals such as personal autonomy or emancipation, but with the means, techniques or skills that contribute to the efficient operation of the state in the world market and contribute to maintaining the internal cohesion and legitimation of the state." In the parlance of my own provincial government, this is knowledge for "workplace readiness" (Alberta Education 2020). The eugenics hidden within neoliberal schools cuts certain people off from flows of investment knowledge such that they can only access payment knowledge used to service social debt.[4]

Third, and resonant with Moten and Harney's concept of logistics, we can note Guattari's (1996, 150–51) distinction between asignifying signs (part- or power-signs), which work directly on material flows, and the signs of signification, which must pass through consciousness to be effective. These semiotics attach to specific forms of instrumental knowledge, which makes their use unevenly distributed. Signs of signification are made "impotent" inasmuch as action can only mobilise on the expressive rather than the machinic plane. Language must interpellate a subject through meaning (it must pass through consciousness and navigate social codes), and thus does not act efficiently like algorithms that, for example, sort what information we see when a webpage loads based on aggregated profiles of listening habits, and thereby change the conditions of action. These algorithms shape *what* we see and come to believe is real, and thereby solicit and constrain action. Although challenged by a variety of actors (such as hackers), the high priests of info-therapeusis claim exclusive right over this semiotic domain and hide proprietary data and code behind technological and legal firewalls.

To take social media as an example, the technicians, programmers who write code, lawyers, and management who use represented data from this massive surveillance machine to make boardroom decisions all draw from streams of capital money, investment knowledge, and asignifying signs. What counts as knowledge here is that which increases the operational performance of an assemblage: "a sense of efficiency measured according to an input/output ratio" (Lyotard 1984, 88). Elite education is needed to craft and wield the asignifying semiotics of these machines that render *Homo sapiens* into talking heads. Psychology has played its part to hack the human mind such that users willingly feed the machines the intimate and detailed data for which advertisers salivate. The users of Facebook obviously interface with the mixed semiotic of Facebook—a medium of both signifying and asignifying semiotics. But in Marxist terms, we do not *own* the algorithmic means of production. Moreover, after accepting terms and conditions, we become alienated from the data of ourselves, which has become proprietary.

We can postulate a final distinction: between *power* and *payment* speech. Power speech refers to priestly words of power. For example, a Catholic priest performs mass using specific words that, at specific times and places, activate networks of power—"in the name of the Father, the Son, and the Holy Spirit." The power of such words is both immaterial and material; they absolve sins and transform matter, turning bread and wine into the literal body of Jesus. The use of Latin (until 1963) in Catholic mass intensified the arcane power of this speech, and in the Middle Ages, inspired priestly impersonators who would proclaim "hocus pocus" (a passable forgery of *hoc est corpus meum*—"this is my body") to illiterate people to activate priestly power and hopefully extort some coin.

The high priests of neoliberalism brandish their own power speech, techno-speak that only specialised experts can understand and execute (especially financial and technical jargon). Talking heads can imitate this power, but what matters, again, is not only the specificity of speech, but the connections of the machine, what the speech plugs into and makes possible. The streams of capital money, investment knowledge, and asignifying semiotics embedded within institutional forms are sites of enunciation that the talking head lacks. The talking head, rather, draws from the common stock of impotentised speech. Is it possible (for activists, including disabled activists, or those pining for the public sphere) to "hack" social media with payment speech and wrest communication from algorithms? Is it possible to render social media an instrument of dialogue or deliberation with careful use? The payment word may be fierce and even true, and may even forge a few power words, but it's what a machine is plugged into and what it can do that matter, not its truth content. Can talking heads turn algorithmic communication towards other ends? How much of this dream is hocus pocus?

For Wendy Brown (2001), the neoliberal condition is to be caught between technological power and political impotence:

> Moving at such speed without any sense of control or predictability, we greet both past and future with bewilderment and anxiety. As a consequence, we . . . feel a greater political impotence than humans may have felt before, even as we occupy a global order more saturated by human power than ever before. (138–39)

This contrast between power and impotence is what Simon Glezos (2021) calls "Brown's Paradox," and I suggest that it exposes an affective link between the talking head and the troll. Glezos writes that Brown's Paradox gets resolved in various ways: neoliberals pretend there *is* no paradox, only the unwillingness of individuals to submit to "market economies, scientific innovation, and individual entrepreneurship" (21); so-called reactionary movements seek to "aggressively (re)secure the foundations of politics and society" (20). The universal priesthood is, with some irony, both influx and efflux of this paradox. The priesthood is a cause as much as a symptom of political impotence, and yet *still* high priests assure us power will flow through more and better speech. We will return below, with Jodi Dean, to this point of communication masking political impotence. On the other side of the coin, becoming-troll, forming a pact with cynicism and nihilism, is a response to political impotence that often (but not always!) aligns with reactionary movements.

Note that within the high- and low-informational priesthoods there exist internal hierarchies (and notice also that priests can take multiple forms—Zuckerberg can squeeze into a talking head for TV). We are all talking heads, yet still plugged into very different networks of power. Elite talking heads such as Anderson Cooper and Sean Hannity come from backgrounds of immense social power and retain the traditional priestly role that Nimmo and Combs highlight of mediating knowledge between the elite and the populace. Such official talking heads jealously guard their insider knowledge and right to speak for elite powers behind the curtain. The exhibition and mastery of style is necessary to stand out in the priesthood, but not sufficient, since, as with Cooper and Hannity, *who* you know matters far more than how you speak (noting the strong correlation between class and rhetorical style). In the end, the power of the enunciation comes from the connections it draws from and operationalises.

The right to special knowledge and to public speech is precisely what the universal priesthood aims to level. Unsatisfied with the prepackaged information spouted by elite (official) talking heads, people with web access can become their own talking head on, for example, YouTube, encouraging fellow talking heads to "sound off" in the comments or reply with videos of their own. At this stratum of the priesthood where social and economic power has more or less levelled out, working the techno-logics of power becomes essential to increase viewers/followers/brand/power. Held up to this machinic standard of performance, disabled talking heads often break. A good talking head whets specific *appetites*; insofar as disability is disturbing it does not circulate well (except in the modes of mockery, pity, or even titillation).

But despite all the differences between talking heads, each one attempts to execute the basic axiom of neoliberalism: "connect those flows! Faster, faster!" (Smith and Protevi 2018). Talking heads feed and excite communication machines, but what function does this serve in the wider priestly context? I here find Jodi Dean's (2009) analysis of neoliberalism helpful. Dean notes that the internet culture has produced new communication strategies for corporate, institutional, and government agents:

> Rather than responding to messages sent by activists and critics, they counter with their own contributions to the circulating flow of communications, hoping that sufficient volume (whether in terms of number of contributions or the spectacular nature of a contribution) will give their contributions dominance or stickiness. (53)

Within this context, participation in the circulation of information *counts* as action such that officials never have to respond to the content of a message (i.e., a specific critique). Rather, in the logic of circulation, style, speed, and repetition overtake content; truth is what "sticks" in the collective psyche.

The high priests—and the social elite—thus adore the universal priesthood and encourage all to contribute their opinions precisely because it dispels institutional responsibility and at the same time assures the political body that they have "been heard" through calls for continued dialogue. The result is that disembodied and disenfranchised organs spout diverse *perspectives* to keep the flow of information and affect in circulation. High priests stage scripted debates that fit discontinuous "viewpoints" head to head, neutralised side by side on screen where the demand for legibility leaves the problematic inarticulable. High priests give talking heads scant time to reduce complex positions to talking points and then defend them in highly polarised fields with no context.

But style, not complexity, is the point. Talking heads sometimes shout to be heard, so as to contribute to the flow of memic talking points. To cite Dean again, "the use value of a message is less important than its exchange value, its contribution to a larger pool, flow or circulation of content" (27). The style of a message, or *how* it circulates, is here more important than *what* it signifies. This is why talking heads spew sound bites: they are signals meant to cut through the noise, rapid-fire bids for attention working according to a machinic logic. The volume of information flow is so overwhelming, Dean notes, that communication produces diminishing returns. To "have one's voice heard" or to make contact through shock effect requires ever-more-elaborate performances of style that either exhibit *or disrupt* dominant norms. That is to say, flouting established norms is a viable strategy for talking heads to gain and retain privilege. But this performance is delicate: to be read as authentic, fresh, or diverse, nonnormative talking heads have to disrupt norms while not being *too disturbing*, thereby subtending normative privilege.

Dean understands the flux of talk to be symptomatic of the weakening of democracy, not a sign of the arrival of democratic deliberation. Perhaps because I know too well the experience of feigned inclusion while being left outside a conversation, I tend to agree with Dean. In fact, as someone disabled, I see a symmetry between the paternalised and feigned inclusion I have felt from the able-bodied and the experience of "being heard" by neoliberal officials. One experience tunes me to the other, and both feel like a pat on the head, some bullshit, and another pat to send me on my way. The bullshit, to be clear, is the fact that each market actor is equal within the flow of signs. As Dean writes, our information-rich society "presumes that all contributions, all sites, are equal, equally likely to be heard or to make a difference" (28). Thus, instead of levelling the centralised control of information, the universal priesthood has produced the dangerous effect of levelling constitutive differences between subjects of enunciation and therefore drowning out stratifications of power.

Connectivity is the basic right and requirement of talking heads (Zuckerberg 2010), and their duties, which spring from worship, include feeding, fixing, and stroking the communication machine of which they are parts. But this analysis remains too general. To understand the existential and political stakes of this universal priesthood, I detail two specific functions of the talking head: passing order-words and smoothing.

Passing Order-Words

The idea that an individual never speaks and that every utterance is shot through with a plurality of voices is probably intuitive to some yet foreign to others. Yet it comes into focus when we consider the talking head's basic function of passing along order-words. Last chapter I skipped across the notion of the order-word in the context of producing the minimal conditions of communication, but now we need to return. For Deleuze and Guattari, an order-word is a prescript—a command that regulates what can be thought and done. They use the example of the teacher, who does not transmit information, but "imposes on her students semiotic coordinates" (1987, 75) that individuate subjects and assign to them social roles, functions, and identities. This marking is called "insigning." In a later interview, Deleuze (2006, 320) explained that "[w]hen you are informed, you are told what you are supposed to believe. In other words, informing means circulating an order-word." Order-words, then, are the stock phrases and ideas that circulate through repetition to prescribe a standardised grammar of what can be thought and done within the world. They are "ready-made ideas, those which are most easily expressed in words" (Olkowski 1999, 90). In this sense, while the teacher insigns, the talking head supplements this function of prescribing pre-made problems and pre-made cures early on.

David Savat and Tauel Harper (2016, 99) suggest that from a Deleuzo-Guattarian perspective, the *purpose* of broadcast news is to modulate desire, to have a strong daddy tell the facts straight (ordering the world) and a mommy comfort us and whisper that, although we don't understand, it will be okay. Order-words simplify the flux of information, offering a frame that reduces ambiguity to make information palatable. Newscaster talking heads draw readily on order-words to frame and make instantly understandable the complex tangle of world events, and YouTube talking heads proliferate memes to cultivate a specific mood, and pundit talking heads repeat "talking points" they have been given to drive home, through repetition, commands about how we ought to understand the world and our place in it. Stated generally: a basic function of any talking head is to speed the flow of order-words.

The meme is the incantation of the talking head.[5] A good talking head will disguise its function of passing along order-words since the order-word is an instance of indirect discourse (i.e., we only pass on what we have heard). A good talking head must still act *as if* they were the subject, the source, of the enunciation, who just happens to be backed by a generic multitude. The subject of communication—the individual who speaks—is for both Deleuze and Guattari always an abstraction from the plurality of enunciative sources. It is not "I" who produce my speech but the "multiplicities, masses and packs, peoples and tribes: all collective arrangements which are within us and for which we are vehicles, without knowing precisely what those arrangements are" (cited in Lazzarato 2006; but see note).[6] Professors are talking heads especially prone to claim speech as our own. But, being honest with myself, much of what I say is simply passing on another's words that are packed within me. Sometimes, I too hunt for talking points that tell me what to think of breaking news. I too often desire to have my world ordered and soothed by Oedipal talking heads.

Sloppy talking heads threaten to expose this mundane function of passing along order-words. When pressed to defend his words, the forty-fifth US president, for example, refused to be subject to his own enunciations and insisted, through repetition, that he was just saying what "many are saying." Talking heads enter into such codependent relationships with order-words because ready-made ideas in the form of clichés, stock phrases, talking points, slogans, or other sound bites are readily intelligible and resonate most widely. But this cuts both ways, since the talking head becomes ensnared by the ordering word; what can be said or thought—what can be problematised—is limited by the common stock of easily expressible ideas. In its functional capacity to circulate order-words (and be rewarded in the form of likes and shares), the talking head thus detaches itself from a self-relation of truth and begins to sound more troll-like.

Communication machines, once again, add their own force to this mix—producing their own orders that constrain what can be seen and heard. We can recall Bill Clinton's training to say everything on a particular topic in less than ninety seconds. What words make the cut? Lazzarato (2016) explains that when preparing for a TV interview, one has in mind ideas about what to speak. Even though these ideas are the product of multiple forces, one still believes oneself to be the subject, the author, of the enunciation. However, television de-individualises the subject: it "functions through the use of a small number of established, codified statements, statements of the dominant reality; it also uses a series of prefabricated modes of expression." In other words, the television machine has other orders, other ideas about what it wants to say, and, through the power of info-therapeutic priests, selects from, interprets, and standardises the interviewee according to "a certain rhythm, certain gestures, a certain mode of dress, a certain colour scheme, a certain setting for your interview, a certain framing of the image, etc." (Lazzarato 2016).

The result, Lazzarato writes, is that we believe ourselves to be the origin of our statements, but we are in fact spoken *by* the communication machine. The more one interacts with such machines, "the more you abandon what you actually wanted to say, because the communicational devices disconnect you from your own collective arrangements of enunciation and draw you into other collective arrangements" (2016). I suggest that this insight constitutes an underlying thesis of the chapter as well as the entire book. What ecologies are these communication machines tearing us from, and what crip ecologies of communication might we instead co-create and inhabit? This is not to deny becoming-machine, but to engage techno-logics in a response more faithful to our irreducibly ecological relations.

Smoothing Machines

Although the concept of smoothness lurks throughout this book, we are now in a position to address it directly and understand the conceptual pair of smooth and striated not as states, but as becomings. "What interests us in operations of striation and smoothing," write Deleuze and Guattari (1987, 500), "are precisely the passages or combinations: how the forces at work within space continually striate it, and how in the course of its striation it develops other forces and emits new smooth spaces." The *smoothing* of striated space; the *striation* of smooth space. Note that striation at its limits can "reimpart" a smooth space. Navigation and cartography striated the once-smooth and chaotic ocean to produce grids that could locate and identify. "This," explains William Bogard (2000, 285), "is the social in its rigid, stratified form, the space of surveilled bodies, bodies that know their bearings." Assigning identities is the most important work of subjection, since, like the ocean, the individual is an organising grid. Yet pushed to its limits, striated space gives way to the smooth. The sea becomes smooth again, "but, in the strangest of reversals, it is for the purpose of controlling striated space more completely" (Deleuze and Guttari 1987, 480). Bogard offers the examples of the submarine that escapes detection by rigid command and control systems and the cyborg that through info- and bioengineering escapes the organism into immortality.

Technologies of info-therapeusis both smooth and striate—these operations are not opposed but always in passage, expressed in mixture. In its striating mode, SLP, for example, organises and identifies subjects within hierarchies of knowledge and power. As I argued in chapter 2, nineteenth-century elocution viewed "proper speech" as a distinguishing *marker* (of humanity, education, social class, whiteness) that produces endless divisions that feed directly into eugenic machines.[7]

But while it striates, it also smooths: SLP machines the semiotic body so it functions optimally in society—smoothing not just the body directly, but its potential for contact with other bodies. It manages not just how one speaks, but the virtual potential to connect parts in a tight "fit." I here consider info-therapeusis to render fluency and its production a matter of *surface contact*, and thus operate as what Bogard (2000, 269) terms "smoothing machines." He explains that smoothing occurs at the interface of heterogeneous spaces, temporalities, bodies, materials, and forms. Society is the production of such machines that assure a tight "fit" between its parts: "No rough spots, no bottlenecks or pinch points, just everything free, clean and fast" (269–70). Dysfluency is one such frictive point that impedes the potential for fast connection. This means, first, that smoothing machines such as SLP unfold interiority to clear a level plane, a maximal yet smooth surface of semiotic contact where the concern is not representation of content but the optimisation of the interface or external point(s) of contact between heterogeneous surfaces. As Paterson (2012, 170) notes, the primary function of SLP is to help dysfluent people "get into" social interaction. And second, we can notice by attending to striation-smoothing that while "proper speech" marks subjects within hierarchies according to class, race, sex, etc., this act simultaneously smooths. Proper speech marks and individuates subjects, yes, but in order to "fit" them to their assigned social role with no ambiguity or remainder.[8]

The talking head emerges from a *clearing* of space, time, noise (dysfluency), and interrelation—smooth sailing ahead. This clearing is what enables the fiction of automatic connection. We can note with Virilio (1997, 91) the relation between smoothing and speed, and that advancements in transportation and telecommunications have always been accompanied by the removal of obstacles from the earth, which is "[n]ever smooth enough, never *desertified* enough" (emphasis in original). Whether constructing underground railways or particle accelerators or fibre-optic networks, "a sort of *superconductive medium* necessarily pops up that will do away with any kind of telluric landmark" (134; emphasis in original). The talking head speeds along smooth highways of communication but also reimparts—creates—such space-time.

Beyond both mechanical and humanist speech, the machinic speech from the talking head (ostensibly) produces a "rhizome" or smooth space of potential for things to form new connections. Pushed to its limits, the striated sea again becomes smooth—the submarine escapes identification.

Smooth talkers *can* facilitate new connections and modes of relation, but can just as easily reproduce dominant meanings in the frenzy to connect flows ever faster. What is the talking head but a smooth relay? The circulation of order-words by smooth talkers is itself a smoothing, a levelling of difference under the force of the easily said. The speed and accuracy with which the machinic tongue can discharge its orders are crucial. Emphasizing the impact of a message is consistent with the function of the talking head to circulate indirect discourse, since the *source* of enunciation does not matter, nor, in the end, does the content. What matters is the imprint of signaletic orders. For talking heads, the shock value matters, but *not* the arrival; the order-words imprint, then continue down the street in constant circulation.

The phrase "everything is going smoothly," Bogard reminds us, means everything is going according to plan and nothing has escaped one's grasp (274). This is the mantra of control that middle managers and managers mutter alike. But "everything is going smoothly" is *also* what we tell ourselves when we sense things going sideways. "Everything is going smoothly" is an anxious mantra to soothe—that is, smooth—a broken machine filled with broken pieces.

On reflection, there are at least four dangers of tethering a universal priesthood to the power of smooth-talking machines. The second two we have yet to address. First, this process debilitates body-minds, which, second, intensifies social inequalities. Some body-minds require more extensive info-therapy to become serviceable talking heads. In repairing/rehabilitating their status as talking heads, disabled rhetors (and other minorities) invest in the *possibility* of "being heard," but also, in this act, do self-maintenance on the communication machine—especially its claim to universality. Everything is going smoothly, murmur the paved-over parts. Third, a population of smooth-talkers-in-waiting presents a legitimate political worry. "It might well be that words," writes sociologist Hartmut Rosa (2010, 57), "and even more so: arguments . . . have become *too slow* for the speed of the late-modern world." Neoliberalism can arguably remake the world faster than the wheels of rational deliberation can turn, universal priesthood or not. This danger is large, too large for my current project to address (cf. Connolly 2002; Rosa 2010). The fourth, related, danger is where I want to focus. This is the *existential* danger of the troll and what Dietrich Bonhoeffer calls "stupidity."

On Trolls and "Stupid" Talk

The fourth problem is quite difficult to enunciate well, but can be approached via the alter ego of the talking head. While remembering that trolling plays many cultural functions, not all of which are malicious, the most relevant kind for our discussion is the weaponised troll. This is what we might call a "breaking machine." For example, within a machinic logic, Sharma (2020, 175) argues that mansplaining is not careless social etiquette that can be cured "by the marginalized taking their turn at the mic or speaking louder." Rather, its "machine logic is about taking up time as a means to drain another of capacity." Like the mansplainer, the troll (and also, in a different way, the talking head) seeks to drain the capacity of their listeners. The troll makes ridiculous claims to incite a response that will use up a "social justice warrior's" capacity and desire. Or, to take another example, the "Gish-gallop" is the rhetorical strategy of throwing a flurry of arguments against an interlocutor, banking on the overwhelming speed of machinic speech to hide weakness of argument. Several right-wing talking-head trolls have made their careers with this tactic, which overloads—breaks—the limited capacity of already broken receivers. "As storage devices for great amounts of *his* information, the Broken Machine's repositories simply have no more file space. They can no longer compute" (175). The mansplainer, troll, and Gish-galloper thus all use the same tactic of reducing the capacity to perceive, compute, and respond, and in this way function as machinic jammers.

Like the SpeechJammer we encountered in the last chapter, a jammer typically functions at the receiver end of communication. In the military context in which it was developed, electronic jamming is throwing noise at an enemy receiver (like a radio tower) to overwhelm the field with noise and *slow down* the rate at which the human-machine receiver can parse signal from noise. This is also the function of what the RAND Corporation calls the "firehose of falsehoods" that is characterised by "high numbers of channels and messages and a shameless willingness to disseminate partial truths or outright fiction" (Paul and Matthews 2016, 1). As an American think tank, it is no surprise that the RAND Corporation would identify the "firehose of falsehoods" to be an issue of Russian propaganda rather than a homegrown problem. And yet, what are weaponised trolls but cultural electronic jammers? Remember, jammers do not block information, but only slow its speed of reception such that, in a world of real-time news, human receivers never have time to parse truth before the next wave of misinformation hits. This strategy is designed to wear out the capacities of semiotic parts. Jammers break other machines by targeting their constitutive connections.

As such, at the register of the political body and political discourse, the universal priesthood bears witness to one of the most vexing issues of democracy, one that is compounded by a commitment to disability justice: namely, individual voices are not and can never be equal, yet must, on some level, be counted as such. Should the enunciations of the ignorant and informed, the rational talking head and the troll, count equally in public reasoning or discourse? Luther savagely attacked parents who withdrew their children from school (Noll 1994, 37) because he recognised—as did Plato, and as would the US founding fathers—that any democratisation of knowledge creates conditions for the tyranny of ignorance and thus requires a sustained, collective, commitment to what the ancients called a *care of the self*. "A people who mean to be their own Governors," writes James Madison (1865, 276), "must arm themselves with the power which knowledge gives." Yet, while I quite agree that reflexive learning is the condition of sustainable self-governance (perhaps especially in the abstracted sense that comes with a federation or republic), it is also true that neither Plato nor the US founding fathers were much concerned about eugenic implications. How do we square these two commitments? Is it possible to make access to and participation within the flow of information universal without at the same time creating the conditions in which smooth talkers, trolls, bots, and people otherwise ignorant of matters on which they speak level the discursive field?

Let me address head-on the eugenic thinking that overshadows this conversation: "Isn't the problem of stupid talk just a problem of stupid people?" After all, I have noted in this chapter that communication technologies continually adjust the barriers to participation in order to maximise the user base, making it as easy as possible for anyone to "join the conversation." The eugenic problematisation is ready-made and even comes with a ready-made and field-tested solution—weed out the *kinds* of people who infect public reasoning. However, while this dream of solving two problems in one fell swoop continues to hold appeal within the eugenic/fascist imaginary, I argue that it is both impossible and deeply misguided. Eugenic thinking can only produce crude proxies such as "IQ" to standardise difference, an abstraction that is not faithful to biosocial realities but nevertheless insigns only on normate bodies the right to enter public channels and participate in public reason or discourse (the *ostensible* duty of talking heads). Capacities, moreover, are relational, such that drawing any eugenic line in the sand—"'stupid' or 'feeble-minded' kinds of people have no right to public reason"—misses the essence of democratic struggle and the tangle of interpersonal and environmental relations through which anyone enters the political.

Bonhoeffer is a helpful guide into this problem. A Lutheran minister and theologian fiercely opposed to Nazi rule, Bonhoeffer was imprisoned and then executed for his role in the German resistance. The paper "On Stupidity" was written from prison in 1942, and, while his eugenic language ultimately impedes his point, it nevertheless deserves consideration. For Bonhoeffer, "stupidity is a more dangerous enemy of the good than malice" (2009, 43), because while evil can be exposed, reasons are utterly useless against the latter. There are two genealogies of the term "stupidity." One is eugenic, of course, but the other lineage, from which Bonhoeffer draws, is more complex. Stupidity here describes, not innate characteristics such as a threshold of IQ, but an overtaking force that renders people *unwilling* to think or judge in the face of emerging events. In this state, a person could and perhaps should know better, but does not. The ableist imaginary tends to fold these two definitions together, solving the political-existential problem of un-listening and un-thinking with a eugenic line of flight. It is thus not surprising that other disablist metaphors attach to this problem. Bonhoeffer himself writes that under this influence, people are "blinded" and "reasons fall on deaf ears." But the careless use of disability-as-metaphor is itself an order-word that displaces two uncomfortable truths.

First, the existence of un-thinking does not correspond with "intelligence" in any normative sense. Bonhoeffer makes this clear. "There are human beings who are of remarkably agile intellect yet stupid, and others who are intellectually quite dull yet anything but stupid" (43). This is not, he insists, a congenital defect, since "under certain circumstances, people are *made* stupid or [. . .] they allow this to happen to them" (43, emphasis in original). Second, recognising this lack of correspondence opens the frightening possibility that the difference is existential. That we can *desire* the order-word even at the cost of believing our own eyes and ears (Orwell 2008, 84) is a terrible thought. Consider the adage—which we often attribute to Mark Twain, but like all indirect discourse, has mutated from untraceable origins—that a "[l]ie will go round the world while truth is pulling its boots on." What accelerates the lie but impedes truth is not, in the end, the technological contraction of space-time (as afforded by platforms such as Twitter), but an existential contraction. Why, in other words, do we desire the lie? The easily said? The ready-made problem and cure? The soothe-saying? Why do we desire to be a vehicle for the order-word, and, in the process, to be ripped from our own sites of enunciation? Here, it does not help to search for *kinds* of people. Instead, we can attend to human differences by understanding capacities as processual rather than fixed outcomes.

Bonhoeffer describes the process in which, "under the overwhelming impact of rising power, humans are deprived of their inner independence and, more or less consciously, give up establishing an autonomous position toward the emerging circumstances" (44). Under what conditions do we surrender our inner independence? In Kierkegaardian terms, perhaps a better word for "stupidity" is to be *led into despair* such that we recoil from becoming and instead seek refuge in the act of levelling differentiation. Kierkegaard, Ada Jaarsma (2017, 57) explains, describes this phenomenon using impoverished terms such as "indifference," "spiritlessness," or the desire "to slip happily and comfortably through the world." It is, she continues, to conform entirely to biosocial norms and to reject all singular differences between speakers—*the self chooses not to choose*, and thus not to engage in differentiation. The result of this indifference towards the difference that constitutes becoming is an existential contraction: "In conversation with him," writes Bonhoeffer (2009, 43), "one virtually feels that one is dealing not at all with him as a person, but with slogans, catchwords, and the like that have taken possession of him." Bonhoeffer captures almost too perfectly the frustration of debating with vehicles for the order-word—that is, either talking heads or their alter ego, the troll. He describes the process of being possessed by order-words as a violent takeover of the self relation, and I would call it a coup d'état save for the fact that we more or less consciously surrender our autonomous position of self-becoming. So yes, the emperor may be naked, but the priesthood is possessed.

What matters for both Jaarsma and myself are the existential affordances embedded within yet exceeding practices of design—for example, the classroom can either level existence to a (pre-set) disciplinary norm *or* spark passion and becoming, depending on the micropolitics of design. Similarly, perhaps the issue of "stupidity" is best considered a matter of design located within a wider collapse of environmental, social, and mental ecologies (Guattari 2000). Here, the problem is strategic erosion, since talking heads are *designed* "to do without thinking, to feel without emotion, to move without friction, to adapt without question, to translate without pause, to connect without interruption" (Moten and Harney 2013, 91) in sterile ecologies that reward split attention and the easily-said.

Social media are a potent example of biopolitical techniques that cut us from the milieu of the problem and then incite cheap talk. Testifying before the US House Committee on Energy and Commerce in 2020, Tim Kendall, former director of monetization at Facebook, highlights the toxicological impact of the machine he helped create. In the same way, Kendall explains, that Big Tobacco expanded their user base with additives such as sugar and methanol (that allow smoke to be held longer) or ammonia (that increase the speed of the nicotine hit), so has Facebook deployed its own toxicological strategies to maximise the contact of attention:

> Tobacco companies added ammonia to cigarettes to increase the speed with which nicotine travelled to the brain. Extreme, incendiary content—think shocking images, graphic videos, and headlines that incite outrage—sowed tribalism and division. And this result has been unprecedented engagement—and profits. Facebook's ability to deliver this incendiary content to the right person, at the right time, in the exact right way . . . that is their ammonia.
>
> [. . . .] When you see something you agree with, you feel compelled to defend it. When you see something you don't agree with, you feel compelled to attack it. People on the other side of the issue have the same impulses. *The cycle continues with the algorithm in the middle happily dealing arms to both sides in an endless war of words and misinformation*. All the while, the technology is getting smarter and better at provoking a response from you. (1–2; emphasis mine)

The problem of mental ecologies is thus toxicological. So yes, we probably need tighter regulations around social media, since *exposure* to misinformation can debilitate a subject very quickly. But the toxin is not simply misinformation, but the very temple of the universal priesthood: less an agora and more a content farm that habituates a restricted capacity to perceive, judge, and communicate.

It is true that right-wing trolls do not have a monopoly on jamming. "Culture jamming" refers to the practice often undertaken by leftist activists (especially in the '90s–'00s) of disrupting the messaging of official channels by subverting the meaning of order-words such as corporate advertising or state propaganda. The phrase was popularised by Mark Dery in 1993 to describe information activists who "introduce noise into the signal as it passes from transmitter to receiver, encouraging idiosyncratic, unintended interpretations." There is something interesting and intuitively right about the strategy Dery offers. Playing at the level of signs to interrupt a monolithic meaning (an order word) can mobilise political energies. And, to their credit, surviving culture jammers such as Adbusters or the Yes People recognise that "hacking, slashing, and sniping" (Dery [1993] 2010) at the level of signs is never a sufficient strategy to enact social justice. The Adbuster's "FUCKITALL Manifesto" is worth stating in full:

> We clean up the toxic areas of our mental environment
> . . . make the price of every product tell the ecological truth
> . . . reverse the upward flow of wealth
> . . . punish every corporation that betrays the public trust
> . . . make secrecy taboo
> . . . bend the straight line in a wobbly new direction
> . . . discover new ways to live, love and think. (BlackSpot Collective n.d.)

Each of these principles resonates with a crip politic. There is a difference between the trollish machine designed to break others and the interruption machine that "bends the straight line in a wobbly new direction." However, I remain convinced that subverting signs has only limited power to revive toxic ecologies in which the talking head and troll flourish. At some level, even the critical action of adding noise to the system is still performing the most basic priestly service for the communication machines: the influx of data that algorithms scrape, process, and use in unimaginable ways. Don't feed the troll! Don't feed the machine!

Bonhoeffer makes clear that only an "internal liberation" can free someone from manufactured despair; no instruction or rational dialogue—that is, talk—can overcome the collapse of inner independence. But even this internal liberation, he concludes, is most often possible only after an external liberation. The existential and political thus figure each other in complex ways that make eugenic solutions to the problems of public reasoning woefully insufficient. What we need instead is a more careful reflection on the political and existential affordances of information access.

Universally Designed Lines of Flight

Deleuze and Guattari (1987, 500) end their discussion of the smooth and striated with a warning: "[n]ever believe that a smooth space will suffice to save us." I want to reflect on this warning in light of Universal Design (UD). Both assistive technologies and practices are, in one sense, smoothing machines.

Whether technical devices such as motorised wheelchairs, which physically intervene in material flows like bodies and sidewalks, or ASL translators who form assemblages with deaf folks, accessibility *desediments* territories that delimit the possibilities for disabled people. In the '70s, crip activists in Berkeley literally smashed curbs with sledgehammers and poured curb cuts under cover of dark. Aimi Hamraie (2017, 240–41) explains that this act has become mythologised in the US disability community such that when activists in the '90s made demands for access to telecommunications that coalesced around the principles of UD,[9] they adapted the history of curb-cutting explicitly. "We have come to the 'curb-pouring' stage in building the information superhighway," announced the vice president of the Universal Access Project. Designing for disability in advance, she continued, will avoid "costly retrofits" to informational systems (cited in Hamraie 241). Electronic curb cuts function as on-ramps to the current of information for blind, hard of hearing, deaf, and dysfluent folks.

Such cuts in material design take nonuniversal embodiments into account; they fold the nonuniversal into the universal through principles of design such as "flexibility in use," and thus produce lines of emancipatory flight, smooth, though prone to capture. Universal Access and Design, in this way, can be a "war machine" (Deleuze and Guattari 1987, 351) that breaks down hierarchical barriers to participation. Goodley (2007) suggests that smoothing can open lines of flight from the delimiting strata of the organism. Becoming-smooth can be a means to escape detection, "to find hiding places, subterranean regions or plateaus, high flat expanses to wander" (153). Access to information, blogs, YouTube channels, and other social media has enabled crip voices to find work, to create community and culture away from overt disciplinary gazes. Autistic culture has flourished online where non-face-to-face and nonverbal interaction are facilitated. Text messaging has impacted deaf and dysfluent communities in similar ways.

But we should note that Hamraie distinguishes two types of curb cuts—liberal and crip—that correspond with either smooth or frictive modes of world-building. The crip activists in Berkeley mobilised *friction* to build access, highlighting—under the cover of dark—the agonistic relations between competing forces in the world. However, "[o]nce integrated into the urban fabric, the curb cut became a material device for securing the place of disability in public space, as well as a metaphor for the *smooth integration* of misfit users into social, economic, and material life" (2017, 97; emphasis mine). Hamraie explains that in the liberal narrative of wide and smooth curb cuts, access is beneficial for "everyone" (wheelchair users, parents with strollers, and skateboarders alike), such that the liberal curb cut heralds a world without friction, without barriers, and thus without disability (2017, 97).

What I find especially useful about Hamraie's analysis is the insistence that curb cuts are "politically, materially, and epistemologically adaptive technologies" (99). The liberal narrative separates the material intervention of the curb cut, the *artifact*, from its political and epistemological intervention such that the *process* of access (its knowledge and making) is left to experts who can maximise smooth inclusion. As such, a central tension for Hamraie concerns "the friction between liberal demands for compliance, productivity, and assimilation and radical, anti- assimilationist, and crip methods of knowing-making the world" (99). The liberal narrative smooths over the very process of knowing-making the world *and* disability as a critical site of this action.

This chapter was framed around the "spectacular accident" of universal access to information being at once a mechanism for disability justice and an incubator for trolls and talking heads. Having arrived on the scene, we find evidence of smooth lines and friction everywhere. When Tim Berners-Lee invented the World Wide Web in 1989, he emphasised its potential for universality due, in part, to his own "frustration with the 'hassle' of using the internet" (Ellis and Kent 2011, 79). Of course, disability must be scaled to reach the summit of the universal. His oft-cited quote is worth repeating: "The dream behind the Web is of a common information space in which we communicate by sharing information. The power of the Web is in its universality. Access by everyone regardless of disability is an essential aspect" (1997). I suggest that Berners-Lee articulates more than a liberal narrative of smooth inclusion for "all" human citizens. More fully, this is a neoliberal narrative of *machinic* inclusion that allows components access to information if and only if they increase the power of the network. Disability scholars Katie Ellis and Mike Kent (2011) write:

> Facebook embodies Berners-Lee's vision where people can share information by reading and contributing. Berners-Lee envisioned the web as a network and recognized that networks become more powerful when more people become members. He saw universal access as a critical component to the success of the web as a network. Facebook is likewise based on the notion of networks as people connect to read and contribute information. It makes little sense to exclude an entire group from independent participation in the network. The Facebook network gains value for each additional member. (104–5)

From the perspective of smooth machinic belonging, disabled populations are doubly productive: not only a sizeable user base to maintain a healthy network, but producers of expert knowledge about adaptive technologies that can be used to benefit "everyone." What drops out of this picture is disability as a site of noncompliant knowing-making.

It is no surprise that disabled people have long considered communication technologies the promise of a better world. When Helen Keller visited Bell labs in 1949 she was transfixed by the curative possibilities:

> Everything I saw at the Bell Laboratories bespoke the civilization to which Dr. Bell looked forward that would unite mankind in one great family by the spoken word. It is true, we are still far from peace despite wider, more swift communications [. . .]. If we only use the advantages worthily that cybernetics is placing within our reach, science will, I am confident, elucidate to us relationships more marvelous than any we have yet comprehended. (303)

With both Keller and Berners-Lee, there is no question that smoothing machines can be emancipatory.[10] Technologies of power, Foucault reminds us, are always constraining *and* enabling. But the world united by communication and mutual understanding that Keller desires sounds too much like our society of control, of mass surveillance and instrumental communication. With Deleuze (1990, 175), "[t]he quest for 'universals of communication' ought to make us shudder." Just as Bell's vision was deeply assimilationist and eugenic, so, in Keller's terms, can humankind only be united "in one great family by the spoken word" through the political establishment of a dominant (or major) language. That is to say, through the oralist demand that we *speak*; ableist norms that police intelligibility; the neocolonial expansion of English; a demand for purity that overcodes complex voices (Lugones 1994; Lugones and Spelman 1983); eugenic practices that screen disability from the world; logocentric prejudices formalised in technical protocols that reduce dysfluency and ambiguity to noise; the circulation of order-words; etc.

Keller's concession is familiar. While faster and more widespread communications *had not yet* created understanding and peace, she maintained hope in the undetermined future when, if we are worthy users of cybernetics, science will reward us with "relationships more marvelous than any we have yet comprehended." Keller would have been dazzled by the garments and trinkets of the universal priesthood. And although she was embedded in eugenic thinking that limited her imagination, Keller would probably be impressed with assistive technologies that enable many disabled and deaf people to participate meaningfully in world-building. I venture to argue, however, that the majority of these changes are extensive rather than intensive. That is to say, the relations of communication, while multiplied and extended, have arguably not grown more marvellous but rather operational and reductive as neoliberalism continues to grind the potentiality of human intra-action into human capital. The promise of cybernetics has soured—despite our service and adoration we are but flickering component parts (Sharma 2020, 177), not the high priests or even gods we desired.

Yet the (neo)liberal narrative continues to taunt: *believe that a smooth space will save us!* In step with its erasure of all social bonds, neoliberalism disavows the very relationality of communication—reducing it to an info-therapeutic problem with technical fixes. To top it off, smoothing machines like Universal Design erase their tracks, rendering the *process* of access invisible and thus unremarkable.[11] This has significant implications for disability politics. Neoliberalism of course recognises that communication is an assemblage insofar as profit can be made through electronic curb-cuts when their production and use can be easily captured by capital. Yet when we cannot recognise the *political* assemblages of communication within which technical assemblages of the talking head always exist (and serve), the complex relations mediated by information technologies become unintelligible and even anathema. There is no space left to politicise and critically appraise messy practices of communication such as, for example, "facilitated communication." We cannot even imagine the enunciation as a co-production. All that is left are clean relations to be managed by the seemingly value-free expertise of info-therapeusis that declare: "I can ease all frictions."

The distinction made by Elizabeth Brewer, Cynthia L. Selfe, and Remi Yergeau (2014) between consumptive and transformative access can help us gain traction at this point. "The former," they write, "involves allowing people to enter a space or access a text. The latter questions and re-thinks the very construct of allowing" (153–4). To use a metaphor crudely, consumptive access is read-only access. Disabled people are here encouraged to be consumers of communication and info-therapeutic technologies under the wide banner of inclusion, but never equal partners in defining "communication," for example, let alone its equitable practice. Transformative access would accordingly include read, write, *and* execute permissions; it is the capacity of those affected to participate in redesigning the rules of the game and thus engage in critical knowing-making of the world. Of door number two, neoliberalism does not speak.

UD is nevertheless a vehicle for both consumptive and transformative access, both liberal and crip practice. Yes, neoliberalism has commodified UD to sell to institutions as yet one more order-word that captures through standardised practice a "static present" (Jaarsma 2017, 144). Dolmage (2016) explains that in this uncritical mode, it is highly possible for UD to

> simply become a proxy system for demanding the flexibility of bodies, increasing the tenuousness of social and physical structures, rebranding our intellectual work, constantly moving the target for technological innovation as flows of information are made ever more proprietary and placing the privilege of "design" in the hands of a narrowing and exponentially profiting few. (111)

The smooth and potentially revolutionary space of UD gets captured by market rationality: becoming another cure for disability, another function of flexibility, efficiency, and profit. Here, UD is most concerned with how to capture the nonuniversal within design; how to increase the consumer base through easy-to-use and flexible interfaces. Market rationality thus limits the neoliberal concern for electronic curb cuts. This is why building on-ramps to information highways is conceivable, but not off-ramps. Why build off-ramps when there is no destination? Why create vacuoles of attention and communication? On the other hand, a commitment to UD in the mode of transformative access is a commitment to self-reflexive design. Transformative access does not call for users, but *co-conspirators* who smash curbs and engage in the process of redesign. Hamraie is clear that the interruptive work of crip technoscience must continue. While consumptive UD privileges the smooth and flexible subject who can adapt at will, transformative UD would ask why flexibility must be so rigid. While consumptive UD makes the public stage universally accessible, transformative UD would mobilise friction to ask who the stage, even the *idea* of the stage, is still working for.

By highlighting the ongoing and collaborative process of design, transformative access returns us to and helps us think through the problematic of public reasoning. Extending a critique of neoliberalism resonant with Jodi Dean's, Brown (2015, 128) argues that "while inclusion and participation are certainly important elements of democracy, to be more than empty signifiers, they must be accompanied by modest control over setting parameters and constraints and by the capacity to decide fundamental values and directions." To be more than order-words that, Brown explains, neoliberalism weaponises against the demos, signifiers such as "inclusion" and "participation" (like "dialogue" or "access") must come with some ability to contest—that is, transform—fundamental values and directions. Otherwise, it's just cheap talk. The worry I have expressed throughout this chapter is that the neoliberal info-therapeutic regime has separated and enclosed these two streams (one powerful, one impotent), then papered over the differences to capture desire within a universal priesthood of infinite contact.

For Jaarsma (2020, 19), the danger of UD lies in subtending pre-set (transcendent) conditions about the world, rather than allowing for and responding to emergent (immanent) actualities. We might need smooth spaces, but they are never sufficient to save us. Info-therapeutic solutions take refuge in universals and smooth over the rough, frictive ground where singular relations could be forged. The problems of information access and the erosion of the demos are thus linked through reflexive design. "When," Jaarsma writes, "we take care to note the structures at play in our methods, such as the grammar of our linguistic scripts, we can notice what is and is not expressed within these structures—and we open up the great array of possibilities that could, in fact, be expressed" (22). These are, ironically, possibilities the talking head can never speak.

Four

Stuttering Parrhesia

In this final chapter, I turn to the issues of political action that the dysfluent speaker, the talking head, and the troll raise. Historically, these issues are not exactly new. With the entrance of democracy, the ancient Greco world faced a crisis of truth-telling; what Foucault (2001) calls a "parrhesiastic crisis." For the Athenian aristocracy, political parrhesia—its semantic range including honest, frank, free, open, and courageous speech—was the civil duty to speak the truth for the good of the populace. The paradigmatic *parrhesiastes* was one who rose before the assembly, staking themselves and their life to an enunciation of truth to power. However, the rise of democracy flooded the assembly with citizens and political voices. With everyone given access to the stage, could the voices of the truth-tellers be recognised? Many feared parrhesia would succumb to the reproduction of flattery, common opinion, and negative parrhesia (ignorant outspokenness) (2001, 66–72). These worries ring familiar, for neoliberalism has produced its own parrhesiastic crisis with a deterritorialising flood of information. Is parrhesia even possible in a field of voice depoliticised yet overrun with market values?

Vignette 11: "Fifteen Million Merits"

In this early episode of *Black Mirror*, a dystopia plays out in large enclosed environments where people run treadmills (while entertained by wall-to-wall screens) to power their habitat and earn "merits" to spend on meaningless shit (Brooker and Huq, 2011). There is one slim chance for escape. The winners of the competition show *Hot Shot* can trade their slavish existence for slightly more autonomy and luxury.

At the climax, the protagonist, Bing, forces himself onto *Hot Shot* with a shard of glass to his neck and something to say. With a ragged voice that shakes with intensity, he indicts not only the judges but also the desire of the audience itself in his critique of the system. "Fake fodder is all that we can stomach. . . . Show us something real and free and beautiful, you couldn't. It'd break us, we're too numb for it, our minds would choke." As his final "fuck you" ebbs, the Simon Cowell clone beams and the crowd roars. "You're right. Authenticity is in woefully short supply. I'd like to hear you talk again." After a moment of uncertainty, the scene cuts and we end in Bing's spacious new house as he films his next allotment of authentic content. Another knife-to-his-neck episode, another channel for the treadmill riders to skip through.

Vignette 12: Shitting in the Street

Diogenes of Sinope, the ancient Cynic, once addressed a crowd extolling the virtue of the great Greek hero Heracles, who took to cleaning a stable full of shit before his death. Diogenes was explaining that Heracles did not *stoop* to this task but performed it with proper dignity since "he considered that he ought to fight stubbornly and war against opinion [*doxa*] as much as against wild beasts and wicked men" (Dio Chrysostom 1932, 397). Diogenes sees the crowd approve of his message without understanding and so performs a live demonstration. He squats and shits on the ground.

• • •

The scene from *Black Mirror* haunts me. Yes, its commentary on informational societies is a little on-the-nose, but it strikes at a deep problem for which I have very few answers. Namely, is it possible to speak truth without its immediate capture? Is it possible to produce ruptures that neoliberalism cannot patch? Recall the quote that opened this book: "Maybe speech and communication have been corrupted. They're thoroughly permeated by money—and not by accident but by their very nature" (Deleuze 1990, 175). Critical theorists cite this line quite often, yet less its immediately preceding context. Negri had asked if control societies might breed a new form of resistance that opens noncapitalist worlds. Deleuze was cautious: maybe, he suggests, "[b]ut it would be nothing to do with minorities speaking out" (175). If speech is a conduit for capital, "speaking out" merely adds to the productive circulation of opinions and perspectives without transforming the underlying conditions. Info-capitalism co-opts the capacity to "speak out" by *soliciting* these impulses at higher and higher levels of deterritorialisation with ever more context-free voices included in the overstimulating discussion: one more viewpoint to be managed as a component part in a semiotic machine.

All these worries of truth-telling amidst global crises roost heavy on my stuttering tongue. Once reduced to a talking head, one can at best aspire to be a sound bite. What truths can be stuttered in this context?

Yet I want to suggest that while these two vignettes, the acts of both Bing and Diogenes, appear the same, they differ in crucial ways. Both are dramatised acts intended to shock, but while Bing's intensity and authenticity intend to communicate, Diogenes's act *exits* the politically inscribed realm of communication. Let me cut to the chase: some types of truth simply cannot be proven as a talking head; some truths cannot be easily said; some truths require shitting in the street. For example: "crip lives are lives worth living." Rosemarie Garland-Thomson (2012) terms the conceit that the world would be better without disability "eugenic logic," and argues that it occupies a dominant place in the cultural imaginary. To call out eugenic logic as a lie, to assert that crip lives *are* worth living, is to speak something nearly unthinkable. Such truths cannot be proven as true in a fight for sound bites, let alone through rational argumentation. Sure, there are good *reasons* to believe refrains like Not Dead Yet or Nothing About Us Without Us or, to take a different example, Black Lives Matter, yet fundamentally, these are not *objects* of knowledge but *rallying cries* in an ongoing critique of power that can only be lived through experimentation. The notion of truth as an embodied practice simply falls flat in the mouth of a talking head.

And yet, the pull to become a talking head is strong. While, for the good humanist, speech takes flight upon the tongue, the crip voice does not discharge meaning like an arrow. Communicating can take embodied effort. Signification must surf our tongues and bodies in a whirl of sounds, gapes, and grimaces. My body is not a docile instrument of reason, but an active participant in signification. It possesses its own agency and secretes its own time. It blocks and repeats some words and phonemes more than others such that communication becomes a type of dance navigated with myself, with others, and with the sonorous environment. Words thus have cost and weight for crip voices. Especially after long days, I sometimes consider the embodied and social effort of asking a question over being silent, or speaking a certain phrase over another. I often cannot afford even cheap talk, so I pick my words carefully. Does this lack of control amount to an impoverished agency? Does an involuntary voice equal a diminished capacity to engage with the world, transform it, and speak truth to power? The clerics of info-capitalism answer in the affirmative; I lived these axioms for many years before I could articulate them, and still longer before I recognised them as indoctrination used to suppress unruly sites of enunciation.

I have argued in this book that communication technologies and electronic curb cuts are unquestionably generative, enabling disabled people to participate meaningfully in worlds that have been historically closed to them. On the other hand, we must reckon with two facts: (1) many truths cannot be spoken as a talking head, and (2) communication machines tend to conflate all voices together under an artificial banner of equality. Neoliberalism is a co-option machine that grinds truths like climate crisis, neo-eugenics, and white supremacy into ever more "perspectives" that must compete—now neutralised—shoulder to shoulder in the marketplace of ideas with flat-earthers and corporate lobbyists alike. Is critique here possible for anyone, *let alone* those voices (disabled and otherwise marginalised) that struggle to be heard on neoliberalism's ableist and hypercompetitive terms? These questions are hemmed, cut short, by neoliberalism's info-therapeutic mode of government that impels individuals to transform and optimize their own embodied capacities in order to stay competitive as continual "entrepreneurs of the self" (Foucault 2008; Fritsch 2015). Within this info-therapeutic regime, dysfluent voices, coded as deviant/pathological, get problematised as noisy, broken, semiotic components awaiting a technical, biopolitical fix.

To retrieve the power of broken machines, Sharma (2020, 177) insists that "[w]e must begin with the knowledge that new technologies will not simply redistribute power equitably within already established hierarchies of difference." Sharma nevertheless remains hopeful that Broken Machines redistribute power through their very existence. Parts that refuse to function as patriarchy or neoliberal ableism intends are a signal, she writes, of the end of business as usual. Yes, the reserve army of parts is quick to smooth over ruptures, but not always. Where then does the political possibility exist for broken machines? Is it, as Sharma suggests (177), in the gap between breaking down and being replaced? Or is it in the heaps of broken parts now decomposing?

This final chapter seeks both to expand the range of what *counts* as political action for dysfluent voices and to find resources that can generate critical breaks in neoliberal modes of power. I accordingly map four modes of truth-telling within the lexicon of parrhesia: therapeutic, Platonic, mischievous, and Cynic. Therapeutic truth-telling is an apolitical enunciation that indexes a model of authenticity and is limited to speaking truth about oneself and the world in a normalising register. Platonic parrhesia is a form of equality-based political discourse that aims at inclusion. In this mode, the parrhesiastes must fashion their body as a pure vessel of truth to be recognised as such. Mischievous truth-telling is the interruption, truth told on the sly by tricksters. The lower-case cynics (especially the trolls) may claim right over this mode of truth-telling, but the Cynics would protest. As such, Cynic truth-telling, finally, is a radical *embodiment* of critique that seeks rupture rather than understanding. Taking up the motto of the Cynics—"deface the currency"—perhaps dysfluent voices can find resources to "de-face" speech and its mythic power, which has become entwined with capital.

Crises of Parrhesia

Allow me to frame the theoretical and political motivations of this chapter. In his 1983 Berkeley seminar entitled "Discourse and Truth" (published in 2001 as *Fearless Speech*), Foucault defines parrhesia as

> a kind of verbal activity where the speaker has a specific relation to truth through frankness, a certain relationship to his own life through danger, a certain type of relation to himself or other people through criticism (self-criticism or criticism of other people), and a specific relation to moral law through freedom and duty. (19)

Foucault takes the ancient model of parrhesia—the exact coincidence between belief and truth, action and speech—to be impossible in the modern socio-epistemological framework. What most interests him is rather the specific *relation* the speaker constitutes with the truth, with others, and thus with themselves in the very act of speaking. Unlike the online troll who attacks behind anonymity and firewalls, and unlike the model teacher who disseminates knowledge of *techne* but risks nothing personal in this relation to truth, the parrhesiastes must summon courage to speak truth in the face of danger about, in McFalls and Pandolfi's terms, "individuals and situations in their ethical singularity" (2014, 173–74). Parrhesia is thus critique; it necessarily takes place within and alters an asymmetrical relation of power. It creates difference in a field of equality—opening a space of danger, hostility, and in some instances even death.

The advent of Athenian democracy buttressed the institutional right to parrhesia with guarantees of both *isonomia*, "the equality of all citizens in front of the law," and *isegoria*, "the legal right given to everyone who speaks his own opinion" (Foucault 2001, 72). Held together, these rights posed a problem: who in this context is entitled to exercise parrhesia? *Isonomia* and *isegoria* in themselves cannot distinguish knowing truth from speaking truth. The democratic crisis of parrhesia emerges when equality without differentiation becomes the ruling political axiom. "Democracy by itself," writes Foucault, "is not able to determine who has the specific qualities which enable him or her to speak the truth. . . . And parrhesia, as a verbal activity, as pure frankness in speaking, is also not sufficient to disclose truth since negative parrhesia, ignorant outspokenness, can also result" (73). Many, from Socrates to Arendt, have worried that under democracy, truth would give way to flattery, the reproduction of common opinion or *doxa*, and thus *negative* parrhesia. The "crisis" Foucault indicates lies in a general struggle between the political and the philosophical life. Who can speak the truth? Who—to use the language of the machines—is trustworthy?

What the parrhesiastic crises highlight is the impotence of action when governed by the single axiom of equality. Lazzarato accordingly suggests that robust democratic societies comprised of agonistic struggle must have what he (2014) and Foucault (2001) call "ethical differentiation" between subjects. While the Athenian constitution guaranteed the equality of speakers before the law, *isegoria* in itself does not determine who will rise to speak. Put otherwise, one does not engage in parrhesia due to juridical status or formal equality: these are never sufficient conditions of political speech and the struggle for justice. The power to speak the (embodied and always risky) truth comes rather from that specific self-relation of ethical differentiation:

> What effectively makes one speak is *dunasteia*: the power, the force, the exercise, and the real effectuation of the power to speak that mobilizes the speaker's singular relations with himself and with those whom he addresses. The *dunasteia* expressed in enunciation is a force of ethical differentiation because it means taking a position in relation to the self, to others, and to the world. (Lazzarato 2014, 230)

It is this differentiation, Lazzarato suggests, that robust democratic societies require to hold open space for the (agonistic) contestation of central values, such that *dunasteia* is precisely what neoliberalism seeks to neutralise. Without ethical differentiation, "parrhesia" can only draw on formal right and equality in a hollow expression of free speech. By reducing speech to the singular logic of capital and thereby erasing distinctions between speakers under the economic banner of unfettered freedom and equality, neoliberalism has produced another crisis of parrhesia. In a perverse twist, it does so this time not merely by drowning out truth in a sea of equality, but by first disavowing and then erasing through info-therapeusis the very (discursive and material) conditions of ethical differentiation.

Who does parrhesia benefit? Foucault explains that while the parrhesiastes does form a pact with themself in the act of speaking, the ethical and political benefit of parrhesia weighs heavily toward the listener. That is, around centres of power swarm "yes men" who flatter leaders with cheap talk and feed, rather than critique, their worst impulses. Flattery produces inattention, obliviousness, and rage.[1] "Because of his insufficient relation to himself," writes philosopher Leonard Lawlor (2016, 250), "the flattered ruler finds himself dependent on the flatterer and his discourse." Parrhesia—honest and frank speech—cuts through the flattery in order to sever the dependent state of the listener, who will then "be able to form an autonomous, independent, full and satisfying relation to himself" (Foucault 2005, 379). While this effect of "freeing" the listener is important and speaks to Bonhoeffer's call for subjects to establish "an autonomous position toward the emerging circumstances," I am equally interested in the effects of parrhesia on the subject of the utterance. How might the parrhesiastic pact the speaker makes with themself produce new existential refrains and territories?

To work towards this consideration of parrhesia as a possible antidote for both cheap talk and the talking head, it is important to differentiate the types of parrhesia. The crisis, remember, is a question of legitimacy staged between the political and philosophical regimes of truth-telling. Who can be recognised as a truth-teller? It is such, Foucault explains, that from the ancient political parrhesiastic crisis emerge two main traditions of truth-telling that stretch across Western history: Platonic (philosophical and metaphysical) and Cynic (ethical and antimetaphysical). It is important to note that both traditions derive from the common fount of Socrates, and each emphasises a different aspect of the Socratic life. Socrates had no time for cheap talk—with conversation and argumentation he woke people to their ignorance and sparked their ire. His parrhesia engaged in political life only indirectly, preparing other people for the political life by helping them govern themselves and others well. Embodying the truth here is important. The parrhesiastes must know herself, yes, but also match her words (*logoi*) with deeds (*erga*) as a sign of truth-speaking. For Foucault, this harmonic accord between word and deed is what distinguishes Socrates from the Sophists—the masters of political parrhesia—who can speak eloquently on courage but are not themselves courageous (2001, 100). To put this in our context, Socrates is an anti–talking head and anti-troll. Chatty gadfly, yes, but Socrates *stakes himself to his utterance* even to death. This difference will be important below.

From the Socratic parrhesiastic fount spring two traditions. The Platonic seeks to prove itself as true through a life of introspection and reason focused around the imperative to know thyself. In contrast, the Cynic practice of parrhesia seeks to overcome ignorant outspokenness and *doxa* (popular opinion) by pushing the Socratic embodiment of truth to its absolute limits. It is this second line of flight that I find most compelling for disability theory. Before turning to these traditions, it is first helpful to shuffle sideways and examine the most ubiquitous rendering of parrhesia within an info-therapeutic regime: free expression or "authentic truth-telling." Therapeutic governance extends a moralised insistence to be authentic and speak authentically, and this imperative short-circuits and depoliticises any act of truth-telling.

Speaking Freely: Authentic Truth-Telling

> The ssstuttering is the most honest part of me / it is the only thing that never lies / it is how I know I still have a voice, I am still -being heard, I am still here / When I stutter I am speaking my own language fluently / When I sound like this I know my loved ones can find me / this is what I sssound like when I speak for myself / this is what I sound like / this is what I sound like.
>
> —Erin Schick, "Honest Speech"

The slam poem "Honest Speech" went viral in 2014 (at least in the stuttering community) and connected in a deep way with many whose voices have long been a locus of shame and silence. Patrick Campbell, Christopher Constantino, and Sam Simpson (2019, xxvi) write in their introduction to *Stammering Pride and Prejudice* that Schick's "open, direct resistance to social norms and reframing of stammering as [their] voice's 'greatest symphony' and 'the most honest part of me' encapsulates the growing movement of stammering pride." The power of "Honest Speech" comes from Schick's voice that resists both pity and pathologisation with each stutter. It is a scandal on stage.

One line in particular seemed to resonate: "stuttering is the most honest part of me / it is the only thing that never lies / it is how I know I still have a voice." Perhaps this line struck because it draws on parrhesiastic themes that link voice to self in a relation of truth. The consensus in the blog and podcast network was an articulation of what we might call an honesty-as-authenticity model summarised well by Katherine Preston (2014) in *Psychology Today*:

> I was instantly attracted to the idea, to the rallying-cry of [Schick's] words, but there was something about the term "honest speech" that gnawed away at me. If my stutter was the most truthful and sincere

> part of me then what did it mean to try and change that voice? What did it mean for the hundreds of people I knew who sought out speech therapy to speak more easily?

Preston raises valuable questions regarding the ethics of self-transformation: Does "honest speech" mobilise a fixed and same-self relation between voice and self? Can one not transform one's voice? These concerns must ultimately be addressed outside a liberal-humanist framework. For Preston, however, honesty, sincerity, and authenticity are all equated. This framing leads her to the anxious question: "did speaking 'dishonestly' mean covering up your true identity?" (2014). Asked inversely: what voice most *accurately* reflects who I *truly* am?

Authenticity is a thoroughly modern concern, and the moral urgency to "be oneself" can be felt in Preston's words, as can the modern drive to manage the gap between outer self and our inner, true, self with a wide range of therapeutic technologies. The philosopher of medicine Carl Elliot (2003, 32) notes that technologies like speech-language pathology have become "a means of remolding the outer body in conformity with the inner being . . . for a person to achieve her true identity." Preston models this humanist desire for what Elliot calls the "perfect voice," which—shorn of unwanted accents, patterns, or gendered pitches—can reveal, in entirety, one's true self. The voice here functions as a reflection of the humanist self that must be biopolitically legible. As education theorist Maggie MacLure explains (2009, 104), "the humanist voice seems to emanate from a subject who knows who she is, says what she means and means what she says," and it is this presumed *transparency* between voice and self that dysfluency interrupts and the therapeutic seeks to restore.

Practices of self-transformation are politically complex: they can reference and circulate dominant norms, yet can also be an ethical practice of self-relation that *exploits* the breaks in these systems of normalisation. It thus comes as little surprise that these practices do not share universal political goals, even (or especially) within critical feminist communities. To take one example, trans activist Leslie Feinberg proclaims that "We are all works in progress" in hir open call for gender expression (1998). Commenting on this text, Cressida Heyes (2007) suggests that such an emphasis on freedom of individual self-expression evades certain normative questions. Namely, it disallows "important political distinctions between progressive transformations of consciousness initiated from within marginalized communities and disciplining moves that attempt only to reinforce established divisions" (55).

Heyes argues that the discourse and practice of self-transformation need to be supplemented by an *ethics* of self-transformation. I turn to the Cynics because they push to its limits such a critical ethos of the self.

Still haunted by the episode of *Black Mirror*, my immediate concern here is how we bundle practices of truth-telling with info-therapeutic technologies; with the way "honest speech" slips into a confessional mode of normalised truth-telling; with how authenticity is an attentional *style* so easily captured by capital. For Foucault, the moral imperative to be authentic stretches back to the ancient philosophical mandate of *gnothi seauton* ("know yourself"). Christianity, he argues, will twist gnothi seauton into a practice of confession—expressing internal states as the means to access truth in general—augmented by the psy-disciplines in the nineteenth century such that knowing and acting in an authentic relationship to oneself becomes the modern path to happiness and well-being.

McFalls and Pandolfi (2014) note the similarity between the ancient and late-modern technologies of the self: between therapeutic governance and the ancient concern with the care of the self (*epimeleia heautou*). Yet they argue that what makes therapeutic care distinct is both its impersonal and exceptional form. Therapeutic governance "can short-circuit any criticism with the questions: who could be against saving a life? . . . And who could oppose applying the technically most efficient procedure in an emergency" (180–81)? When disability is naturalised (Tremain 2017) and its undesirability prefigured within society (McRuer 2006), therapeutic intervention comes to possess a compulsory and seemingly rational mandate. What kind of person *would* oppose speech therapy for young children with disabilities? As McFalls and Pandolfi note, "[t]o do so would be pathological and justify further therapeutic intervention" (181). In short, while late-liberalism works to enhance the life of the population, this is always according to and constrained by market veridiction. The market restricts the *kinds* of self-practices and truths disabled people can embody and the possible modes of subjectivisation from which we speak. Therapeutic technologies are a means to cultivate one's capital (social, genetic, linguistic, etc.) at the same time as they depoliticise this speculative process, which makes a therapeutic regime fundamentally at odds with the political.

Thus, while disabled people must shoulder the economic and affective costs of finding "the perfect voice," there is no room in the conversation to contest structural inequalities or disadvantages that people with communication disabilities face. All that remains are market realities and unending crises to manage with value-neutral therapeutic solutions. Who *wouldn't* want maximal control over their communicative body and to be understood completely and immediately? What sort of person *wouldn't* want therapy—for either themselves or their preschool child? Such questions posed in an impersonal and exceptional form are meant to close conversation, their answers prefigured by a compulsory and eugenic logic (McRuer 2006; Garland-Thomson 2012). But what if, once again, we took such questions as beginnings rather than endings?

The insistence on an authentic voice generates an impoverished relation to oneself, to others, and to the world. The moralised imperative to be always authentic drives us toward the shoals of same-self identity. Further, authenticity plays within a normalised field always delimited by brand rating that predisposes practices such as "self-acceptance" (typically expressed in a confessional mode) to lean toward fixity of self rather than true self-experimentation. Therapeusis collapses honesty into authenticity, and parrhesia into "speaking freely." This redefinition of parrhesia rings clear in Sara Bareilles's 2013 pop song "Brave," where courage is expressed by *letting* the inner truth *fall* from our mouths. "Say what you wanna say / And let the words fall out / Honestly I wanna see you be brave." But while truth-telling in the therapeutic mode—speaking honestly, freely, authentically about oneself—might be a practice of self-transformation, it will not help us escape "the veridictional cage of the market" (McFalls and Pandolfi 2014, 174). With enough therapy, we might become servable talking heads capable of "speaking out"—but wasn't this precisely Deleuze's worry? What if we take a different approach and imagine (with Foucault) honesty as a mode of *critique* rather than authenticity? We might hear Schick's proclamation that "Stuttering is the most honest part of me / it is the only thing that never lies / it is how I know I still have a voice, I am still being heard, I am still here" as the embodiment of critique rather than a claim of identity.

Pure Vessels of Truth: Platonic Truth-Telling

In this section I suggest that the Platonic mode of parrhesia seeks to overcome negative parrhesia by fleeing rather than affirming the rhetorical body, and thus always and already constructs the disabled body as what Simona Forti (204, 205) terms an impure "vessel of truth." The Platonic tradition (from which therapeutic governance draws) aims to prove itself as true through introspective reasoning to "know thyself." It is such that this tradition engages in what Foucault calls the "analytics of truth" concerned with knowing and recognising true statements (especially of the self), in contrast to the Cynic tradition, which, as I explain below, belongs to the "critical tradition" in Western philosophy concerned with the importance of *telling* and knowing *why* we should tell the truth (Foucault 2001, 170).

One significant point of departure of Platonic from Cynic parrhesia concerns the question of the body: must truth flee or affirm the body in order to overcome the political conditions of error and negative parrhesia? Foucault (2012) explains that the Platonic approach draws from the Pythagorean practice of purification, one that stretches from pre-Socratic into modern philosophy. "The transition from the impure to the pure, from the obscure to the transparent, and from the transitory and fleeting to the eternal constitutes, or at any rate marks the moral trajectory through which the subject can be formed as a subject capable of truth" (125). Disability is one such deviating influence of the body that thwarts reasoned control. A proper subject of disability must, through diligent therapeutic care, constitute themselves as a pure vessel of truth in order to be capable of telling and recognising the truth. The vessel of truth is the sovereign self; with others they converse in a "reasoned, metaphysical convergence of souls" (McFalls and Pandolfi 2014, 175). The Cynics, as I will show, take the quite opposite approach in affirming the material necessities of life. They seek to shock and provoke—to reveal truth and the hypocrisy in common opinion through parrhesiastic displays of the body.

From within the Platonic tradition, disabled people are cracked and untrustworthy truth-tellers. Recall from last chapter that Yergeau (2018, 60) argues that rhetors stamped with "marked and stigmatic presence" are suspended in a "demi-rhetorical" state. The tongue must first be mastered before it can be trusted. Yet if marked as kakoethical—as *bad*—even "successful" rehabilitation might not be enough to secure inclusion within the political body.

In response to such structural exclusion of disabled voices from the realm of rational deliberation, some disability theorists, such as Stacy Simplican (2015), seek to expand the range of voices at the table. Simplican desires to revive practices of deliberative democracy through a "reflexive deliberation" that broadens communicative norms to make space for disabled voices. In the first place, she maintains that physical presence, in the absence of or in supplement to linguistic vocality, communicates the needs of participants. Secondly, Simplican argues for an understanding of speech as collaborative in which deliberative participants can make claims together and thus shore up individual "deficits." For Simplican, unmooring the practice of deliberation from the hegemony of language can greatly expand the range of political participation and the place of disabled peoples within democratic societies.

While I am supportive of such projects, I here want to expand the range of action itself—calling the political stage itself into question. This is not least because I fear that disabled subjects will always be "demi-rhetors" in the space of rational deliberation. The Platonic strategy to transcend opinion and error is, ultimately, to close oneself to the rhetorical body itself: to nature, nonhuman life, and to other forces of becoming-other. Foucault (2012) explains that the Platonic tradition of care aspires towards purity because its ultimate movement (via truthful knowledge of the self) is directed towards the "other world"—a transcendent world of unchanging truth where souls bask in harmony.

Yet the Cynical tradition develops along a different path and models a different politic. As Foucault (2012, 245) writes, the Cynics posed a different question: "[n]ot the question of the other world, but that of an other life (*vie autre*). . . . The other world and other life have basically been the two great themes, the two great forms, the great limits within which Western philosophy has constantly developed." To cultivate an other life—one of radical and embodied otherness—is to seek to change *this* world here and now, not to seek refuge in (or draw from) a metaphysical beyond. This practice engages in what Alexis Shotwell (2016) and other social movement and anarchist theorists call "prefigurative politics": a collective way of acting that reflects and thus enacts the world we desire. To quote Chris Dixon (2014, 84–85, cited in Shotwell 184), "*how* we get ourselves to a transformed society (the means) is importantly related to *what* the transformed society will be (the ends). The means *prefigure* the ends. To engage in prefigurative politics, then, is to intentionally shape our activities to manifest our vision." In the context of dysfluency, one cannot expect to enact a habitable world fluently.

One can, as such, read the history of disability activism as constituted by both questions: the other world and an other life. On the one hand, disabled subjects have had to strive for the "brass ring of normality" (Overboe 2012, 117) and play the part of the detached rational speaking animal to have our truths heard in the most minimal sense. We have had to purify our bodies in the hopes of being more than demi-rhetors. The landscape of disability rights and activism has historically been eclipsed by those (white and often straight) physically disabled subjects who are capable of claiming the status of a talking head, and thus social worth.

The bid for recognition and inclusion in the major grammar has, yes, furthered rights-based legislation and discourse for disabled peoples. Yet it has also meant excluding those who fall outside the bounds of the human linguistic community (guarded by racial and gendered boundaries). It is for such reasons Puar argues (2013, 182) that disability studies must challenge the "status of rational, agential, survivor-oriented politics based on the privileging of the linguistic capacity to make rights claims." However inescapable, the act of composing ourselves as proper disabled subjects—nearly normal!—for state recognition reproduces liberal-humanist binaries (communicative/noncommunicative; worthy/unworthy; rhetor/demi-rhetor) that turn the disability community against itself on the always-deferred promise of the "other world" of Right, Justice, and Equality for all.

But at the same time, one can also read in the history of disability rights the composition of "another life." Artists such as Eli Clare, Sins Invalid, and Lindsay Eales (to name a few) have kindled other ways for crips to exist. And Corbett O'Toole (2015) depicts the communitarian ethos that marked the early days of disability activism at the Center for Independent Living in Berkeley, California, in the '60s. She describes raucous dances and parties as an important feature of social life—bodies marked as deviant or asexual reclaiming pleasure. In this framework, to cultivate an other and unintelligible life might be equally political. The lesson, perhaps, is that equality and recognition are often necessary yet never sufficient conditions of disability justice. To remap the human sensorium, to produce new types and *possibilities* for relation, is not just a care of the self. It is already to alter the world. Let us now turn to Cynic truth-telling.

Mischievous Truth-Telling

I lied. The next stop is not the Cynics but the trolls. Or perhaps, as happens among those with dysfluent speech, I did not lie, but simply blocked on the word "Cynics" and interjected something easier to say. Or perhaps I *am* telling the truth, just not telling it straight. Does it matter which?

To troll or to stutter are both interjections, both interruptions to the regularly scheduled program. The troll jeers at those who wait for their turn to speak at the microphone and breaks norms of rational deliberation to break ~~onto~~ the stage. Recognising the queue itself to be a neoliberal charade, the troll makes a pact with cynicism; it interrupts by exploiting both the precarity of communicative norms (like turn-taking) and those "normies" still bothering with good faith. I too feel the cynicism and largely agree with the conclusion that telling truths "straight" (in queues and official channels; with fluent and authentic bids for recognition) is not *sufficient* when the game is rigged.

Like the troll, the stutter also frustrates a well-ordered queue, it too interrupts norms of rational deliberation. But my argument is that the dysfluent interruption is of a different kind—not an exploitation but, if we are willing, an invitation. I am compelled by Judith Butler's (2005, 91) claim, drawing on Emmanuel Levinas, that "responsibility is not a matter of cultivating a will, but of making use of an unwilled susceptibility as a resource for becoming responsive to the Other." Remember that the SpeechJammer was carried into existence by the utopic/dystopic dream of perfect noninterruptibility. To undercut the unavoidability of speech is to be severed from our unwilled susceptibility to the world—unplugged from our source of responsiveness and thus action. But before following the divergence of the dysfluent and troll too far along, I want to linger in their messy resonance. Namely, both actors speak in the mode of the trickster.

The feminist philosopher María Lugones (1987) argues that there are different modes by which one inhabits one's own world and "travels" to foreign worlds. We find ourselves at ease within a world—"fluent" within a world—due to a combination of factors: linguistic mastery, agreement with social norms, human bonding, and shared histories. However, Lugones warns that being maximally at ease within a world, being *too* familiar, makes it difficult to travel. She thus draws a helpful contrast between *playful* and *agonistic* world-travelling.

Agon means "contest" or "struggle," and in one formulation designates a hypermasculine field of aggression in which we can imagine all sorts of trollish behaviour. "An agonistic sense of playfulness," writes Lugones, "is one in which *competence* is supreme. . . . In agonistic play there is risk, there is *uncertainty*, but the uncertainty is about who is going to win and who is going to lose" (15, emphasis in original). Familiarity within a language game collapses into mastery over, a tight grasp of, its rules and meta-rules. Only the most competent talking heads and trolls win the game of interruption tag.

I agree with Lugones that the agonistic traveller is often an imperialist, the Western conqueror, the Conquistador who makes the world its stage of violent "play"—yet I also believe she dismisses the possibilities of agonism too quickly. The trope of the manly political warrior obscures more interesting ways of agonistic acting-in-relation. In the first place, agon is not, strictly speaking, about winning—Nietzsche (2006) *especially* recognised that agon's existential (and civic) virtue lies in struggle rather than conquest, rendering necessary social restrictions against becoming too strong and thereby collapsing the contest.[2] Moreover, agonistic struggle manifests as a playful *self*-relation that slips through the tight grasp of self-sovereignty. Guattari (2000, 33) implores his readers to cultivate an "internal dissensus," while Bonnie Honig (1993) offers the transgressive figure of the *virago* as a model of agonism.[3] Agonistic action, in other words, does not primarily deal with the actual (e.g., talking points), or the potential (e.g., risk factors), but the *virtual*—those possibilities that might be, if attended to and welcomed.

Instead of the warriors who struggle and ultimately fail to world-travel insofar as they assimilate and destroy the world of the other, Lugones (1987) offers the playful figures of the trickster and fool:

> Positively, the playful attitude involves openness to surprise, openness to being a fool, openness to self-construction or reconstruction and to construction or reconstruction of the "worlds" we inhabit playfully. Negatively, playfulness is characterized by uncertainty, lack of self-importance, absence of rules or a not taking rules as sacred, a not worrying about competence and a lack of abandonment to a particular construction of oneself, others and one's relation to them. (17)

To embody the playfulness of the trickster or fool is not to give up on agonistic relatedness, or for that matter, on rational deliberation. It is to ask for a more robust kind of agonism where sedimented constructions of the self and its place within hierarchies are also up for grabs. The confident troll, of course, already claims a playful territory—"[t]rolls believe that nothing should be taken seriously" (Philips 2016, 25). Yet the differences are obvious. Openness to becoming-fool is far different than making other people into fools! Not taking anything seriously is far different than opening oneself up to such practices in a critical mode, out from a position of anonymity.

Openness to being a fool "is a combination of not worrying about competence, not being self-important, not taking norms as sacred and finding ambiguity and double edges a source of wisdom and delight" (Lugones 1987, 17). This describes the trickster, yes, but also the disabled rhetor, the crip who finds some mischievous delight in mistakes and mucking about language. In *Disability Rhetoric*, Dolmage argues that the Greek god Hephaestus—both disabled and trickster—embodies the rhetorical notion of *mētis*: "the cunning intelligence needed to adapt to and intervene in a world of change and chance" (2013, 50). The feet of Hephaestus twist in opposite directions; he thrives through creative invention, notably of machinic prosthetics. Dolmage reminds us that "[t]ricksters are prosthetic rhetoricians" (219). Hephaestus is cunning *because* he cannot walk straight, making use of whatever can be found with prosthetic and sideways movements.

My point, in short, is that when both troll and dysfluent crip utter their truths, they do so mischievously, and, moreover, that both actors engage in a type of agonistic struggle that seeks to surface and unsettle deep-seated values—not through the content, but the form of the utterance. Both are acts of interruption. Where the truth-telling capacities of the troll and dysfluent crip diverge is the possibility of parrhesia: the *pact* the speaking subject makes with herself in the act of speaking. Foucault (2010) explains that this pact has two levels:

> the level of the act of enunciation and then [the one], implicit or explicit, by which the subject binds herself to the utterance she just said, but binds herself also to the enunciation. . . . On hand the subject says in the *parrhesia*: Here is the truth. She says that she really thinks this truth, and thus she binds herself to the utterance and to the content of the utterance. But she makes a pact as well here as she says: *I am the one who said this truth; thus, I bind myself to the enunciation and I take the risk of all its consequences*. (62; emphasis mine)

On full display these days, the troll, perhaps in good company with the trickster, will not accept either part of this pact. The troll doesn't *really* believe its words and will never be bound by them. It trolls for amusement, for the "lulz," and mustn't be caught caring. I am again reminded of Sartre's (1948, 13) description of anti-Semites who "even like to play with discourse for, by giving ridiculous reasons, they discredit the seriousness of their interlocutors." Yet one need not be "serious" to bind oneself in a double manner to the utterance. After all, seriousness lends itself to a mastery of the world. Serious talking heads utter serious statements, but like the trolls have no need to bind themselves to their enunciations. The pact is a necessary condition of parrhesia. The attempt to utter parrhesia without binding oneself to the enunciation devolves the utterance into outspoken ignorance—indirect discourse that can circulate irrespective of the source of enunciation. "Whoa! *I* didn't write that." "I'm just saying what I heard!" "Can't you tell I was joking?"

Thus, to proclaim with Schick that "[t]he sstuttering is the most honest part of me / it is the only thing that never lies" is not to concede that one can only stutter the truth straight, but rather to affirm the dysfluent body as a parrhesiastic locus. To rephrase Foucault: "I am the singular being who stuttered this truth; thus, my stutter binds myself to the enunciation and I take the risk of all its consequences." Dysfluency, as I argue below, can create existential territories; if we let it, it can re-plug us into sources of shared responsiveness and action. But to do so requires a shift from the head to the anus, from *logos* to mutant subjectivation, from cynicism to the Cynics.

Cynic Truth-Telling: Stuttering from the Anus

Allow me to take stock. In an aggressive manner, neoliberalism has extracted cheap talk from bodies and triggered a triple ecological collapse: environmental, social, and mental. Info-therapeusis is well underway un-terraforming the planet, the socius, and the mind in the service of connection. Each of these modes of collapse works on the others, and each is implicated in the contemporary crisis of parrhesia. Yet without diminishing the importance of the first two ecologies, the crip intervention I, with the Cynics, offer is most concerned with the latter ecology. In other words, without denying the toxicological effects of either information and misinformation on the sociopolitical body, or the structural conditions that make these flows possible, I am drawn to the problematic of the *subject* of the truth-utterance and thus to the existential (what Guattari would call the ethico-aesthetic) resources that the ancient Cynics might offer in response to cheap talk.

Dysfluent speakers will always be deficient—little demi-rhetors—in the Platonic model of action, and I suggest in this final section that the Cynics offer an alternative becoming, a way to speak otherwise that invites "an other life." In contrast to the Platonic model that desires a communion of rational souls, the Cynics take the quite opposite approach by radically affirming the material necessities of life. Peter Sloterdijk (1987) describes Cynicism as "cheekiness from below," which, he explains, means both that Cynicism necessarily embodies power from below—power that punches-*up* against a hegemonic order—and that the embodied critique of Cynicism draws its power not from the head but the ass. Diogenes of Sinope lived contemporary with Plato and would publicly mock the philosopher as well as wider prevailing social norms with dramatic, cheeky, acts. For example, he famously responded to Plato's theory of ideas with a fart, and his theory of *Eros* with public masturbation (101). Diogenes short-circuited the "headiness" of Platonism to present, through his material body, such a challenge to both doxa and philosophy that Plato called him "Socrates gone mad" (102)—quite a fascinating admission from the perspective of critical disability studies. The important point is that his radically materialist and antipolitical parrhesia does not draw from the same sources of power as do Platonic talking heads. "Cheekiness from below is effective when it expresses real energies as it advances. It must consciously embody its power and alertly create a reality that can at most be resisted but not denied" (110). Cynics can stage the possibility of another life, but *only insofar as* they radically do what they say. In other words, the Cynic recognises that some truths cannot be said.

Foucault suggests that ancient Cynicism is the birth of the "critical tradition" in Western philosophy concerned with the act of *telling* the truth and knowing *why* we should tell it (2001, 170). It is such that the Cynics seek to shock and provoke—to transform our perceptual apparatus and reveal truth and the hypocrisy within common opinion through parrhesiastic displays of the body. Instead of participating within popular discourse, the Cynics thus told the truth outside language. They dramatised the mundane reality of life by living exposed, publicly, and without shame. This tradition proves itself (against doxa) by taking the self, and life more generally, as a continual challenge. It scrutinises and experiments with forms of life in order to alter the possibilities and conditions of this world.

Foucault (2012, 218–19) explains that the Cynics prove their way of life as truthful, set against both political and philosophical parrhesia, by turning upside down and pushing to their limits the four Ancient Greek characteristics of the true life. (1) Truth as nonhidden or unconcealed becomes for the Cynics a *scandal* of absolute visibility; (2) a life of truth as unalloyed or without impurity becomes a life of radical poverty and indifference; (3) the "straight" life set in conformity with both *logos* and *nomos* is now judged by the single law of nature; and (4) sovereignty, or a self-mastered and self-fulfilled life, becomes a type of philosophical *militancy* for and against the world. One dominant theme that runs through these reversals is the self is taken as a *site* of continual challenge rather than an *object* of knowledge. Truth manifests through embodied practice rather than argumentation amongst purified souls.

For the Cynics, the true life is revealed in fearless and creative undoing of the self: the continual challenge of absolute visibility, radical poverty, animality—and above all, of shamelessness. The Cynics seek to strip away social conventions and beliefs that, from the perspective of "nature,"[4] are utterly arbitrary. They thus engage in the radical practice of transvaluating values, a motif reflected in their motto "deface the currency" (*parakharattein to nomisma*). Foucault suggests we read this as an imperative to *alter* rather than simply erase the value of the current coin. This reading highlights the link between currency—*nomisma*—and law—*nomos*. To alter the currency, Foucault (2012, 227) writes, is "to adopt a certain standpoint towards convention, rule, or law." The scandalous life targeted those habits, customs, and institutions that conceal the natural law. The Cynics sought to alter the stamp on existence; to give a new form to life that emerges from life itself. This, Foucault writes, is a transvaluation of values, an immanent political project that stages "life in its material and everyday reality under the real gaze of others"

(253). Dramatic acts that transgressed social codes such as eating and making love in public were meant to shock and force others to think, to feel. In the neoliberal context where speech is thoroughly corrupted by capital, it might be a thoroughly political act to change, debase, or alter speech.[5]

Insofar as Cynic truth manifests in the radical affirmation and transvaluation of nature, the body, and its passions, we can understand Cynic subjectivisation as a Deleuzian war machine that destroys territories and barriers like those instilled through shame. Vanessa Lemm (2014, 219) explains that "the Cynics abolish the public/private division by dissolving the immunitary barriers of civilization, thus opening up the possibility for a public life that is truly communal." Shame keeps many people, especially in the disability community, hidden away from public life and from community. The fear of pissed pants, shitting in public, or stuttering uncontrollably before others are real barriers that keep crips "in their place." But such barriers won't be overcome by clawing after formal equality and right. Since the problem is misplaced shame about, for example, shit (i.e., we shame the material facticity of shit rather than shaming such social conventions around shame, the sites where exclusions get reproduced), what we need is a transvaluation of both shame *and* shit.

We might, as a start, consider Daniel Martin's (2016) essay "Stuttering from the Anus"—a remythologisation of stuttering. "In a letter to Sándor Ferenczi from 26 November 1915," explains Martin (123), "Freud writes in passing that stutterers 'have projected shitting onto speaking.'" Put otherwise, adult stutterers are stuck in the anal stage of childhood development and seek to resolve narcissistic conflict by spewing words like verbal diarrhoea. Rather than deny the thingness of speech and the narcissistic pleasure of spewing it around, Martin suggests that stutterers *embrace* words as "excremental remains of embodiment, echoes of the inert involuntary thingness of our bodies prior to that abstract concept we call 'life'" (121). Martin reminds us that the voice does not come from the mouth but always from an uncanny "elsewhere" that we cannot identify, let alone control. (To channel Margrit Shildrick's [1997] theory of "leaky bodies," perhaps the voice is not summoned but *leaks* from bodies in uncontrollable drips and puddles.) In this reading, speech, like faeces, is an unsettling presence, a bodily link to others that reveals our radical intersubjectivity.

> Here's my ultimate thesis for anyone with dysfluent speech: spew your shit. Let your speech stutter from the anus. Don't preach inclusivity, awareness, or acceptance; such weak emancipatory goals are thor-

> oughly infused with pedagogical desires for fluency. A demand for one's voice to be heard is a demand for fluency. Be a constant reminder to anyone who will or won't listen that the voice doesn't just come from the mouth. It's physical, crypt-like, and buried. (129)

With Martin, we must affirm the material and uncanny source of speech if we are to undo the privacy of the dysfluent voice and "blast it into the social" (Martin 2016, 129). And with the Cynics, we must attempt a radical affirmation of life through an ongoing critique of the politics of *shame* in order to challenge the public/private divisions that keep disabled peoples marginalised. What is stuttering from the anus but to mock like a Cynic those talking heads who have crawled far up their own assholes in order to be respectable? Yet this interruption to cheap talk is more than a negative critique; stuttering from the anus is an existential practice that enacts other sources of power and connection.

Before we explore the power of the anus any deeper, it is important to note that shit, faecal matter, is debilitating—toxic to environmental and biosocial ecologies—and sanitation is not equitably distributed. The World Health Organization records that in 2017, two billion people (~27% of the world population) did not have access to toilets or latrines and that 673 million of these would shit in the open (World Health Organization 2019). The differentials flows of shit are a matter of justice and are biopolitical (or perhaps necropolitical), since, as the WHO also notes, inadequate sanitation is linked to malnutrition, reduced socioeconomic outcomes, and the transmission of various diseases such as cholera, dysentery, hepatitis A, typhoid, and polio, and moreover, an estimated 432,000 diarrhoeal deaths per year (2019). Especially for crip theory, the politics of shit is simultaneously a laughing matter and deadly serious. It is such that I seek to follow a long line of theorists and activists (stretching from Diogenes to queer theorists such as Leo Bersani) that recognise the anus and shit to be sites of always impure politics. In the remainder of this chapter I briefly elaborate the notion of stuttering-from-the-anus in the context of three related Cynic themes: animality, the rejection of recognition, and becoming-imperceptible.

First, the namesake of the Cynic tradition (*kunikos*—Cynic; *kuōn*—dog) reflects their shameless affirmation of life. People commonly called Cynics dogs because they lived radically poor and set against social convention, yet nevertheless without shame and with indifference to prevailing opinion. The dog's life is the unconcealed life embodied by *zoe*, "the human being's animality taken up as a challenge, practiced as an exercise, and thrown in the face of others as a scandal" (Foucault 2012, 265). For Lemm (2014, 211), again, to affirm animality is to attack the immunitary devices that divide life from truth, nature from culture, animal from human. To this list I would add those devices that separate noise from speech, the tongue from the face, from the head, from the body. If neoliberal subjects are in danger of becoming talking heads, or automatic connection-machines, to let the stutter come from the anus or at least to "relocate it away from the mouth or the brain where others would prefer it remain" (Martin 2016, 129) is a resolute practice of animality that tells the symbolic, drunk on its power, to go fuck itself.

To return to the second vignette of this chapter, Diogenes squats and shits in the middle of the street when he senses that the organs of his head were mystifying his audience rather than revealing the truth he meant to utter. Lazzarato (2014, 243) suggests that the singular power of the Cynic parrhesiastes to open "an other life" comes from the fact that the Cynics are not "speaking beings" but rather bodies that enunciate through diverse semiotics: "Gestures, actions, example, behavior, and physical presence constitute expressive practices and semiotics addressed to others through means other than speech." Diogenes was explaining that a great hero like Heracles would have no reason to be ashamed getting his hands dirty with shit in a barn. The message is that one considers cleaning stalls to be loathsome only due to common opinion; this labour too is virtuous. (This truth resonates since I grew up below the poverty line and cleaned many very shitty bathrooms over the years before joining the academy, where any serious talk of class is a faux pas.) So instead, Diogenes turns to the "elementary organ" of the Cynic (Sloterdijk 148) to shatter a false consensus and demonstrate that our reasons for shame are out of joint. (For example, perhaps heady professors should be less ashamed of shit and more ashamed of how little janitorial staff get compensated to manage professors' shit and shame.)

Diogenes "literally shits on the perverted norms" (Sloterdijk 168) because the head will never relinquish its respectability. Actions such as shitting in the street are thus enunciations that exit language, a non-discursive rupture, both a test of animality and a cheeky critique of paper-thin consensus like a neoliberal commitment to social "equality." Lazzarato (2014, 243) explains that language for the Cynics carries not merely a denotative and representational but also an *existential* function that "helps construct existential territories." The Cynics participate in *logos* but their speech does more than represent or denote: it gives a form to existence. In this way, the self enacts

> something that runs counter to the "normal" order of things, a counter-repetition, an intensive given which invokes other intensities to form new existential configurations. These dissident vectors have become relatively detached from their denotative and significative functions and operate as decorporealized existential materials. (Guattari 2000, 45)

The abrupt intrusion of ugly objects or part-signs such as dysfluent words into public space holds power, detached from the word's linguistic functions, that can shock and disrupt (ableist) common opinion and sensorial domains. But such intrusions are also "mutant nuclei of subjectivation" (1995a, 18) that can invite new, unexpected, becomings. Insofar as "[s]pirited materialism is not satisfied with words but proceeds to a material argumentation that rehabilitates the body" (Sloterdijk 105), shitting in the street can be an existential practice—not a therapeutic or curative rehabilitation, but one of embodied existential vitality. That is to say, sometimes a self can only grow when planted in shit.

Second, to stutter from the anus is to reject recognition. Unlike other philosophical schools, the Cynics had no interest in proselytising to gain the most followers and thus needing to conform to norms of intelligibility and social propriety. The logic of recognition cannot think beyond the sovereign self: an individual creature—a hierarchy of organs—defined by reason and right. The Cynic life is one of fierce and relentless critique, not of the city or State but the entire world—the body of the Earth. The Cynic life attacks "the conventions, laws, and institutions which rest on the vices, faults, weaknesses, and opinions shared by humankind in general" (Foucault 2012, 284–85). This critique is always first and foremost a work on the self (a creative undoing, the formation of what Deleuze and Guattari would call a Body without Organs). The struggle for the stutterer is not "to be heard" or to be recognised as a talking head, but to transform the constellation of (human and inhuman) forces that produce and fix the identity of "disabled speaker" within an info-therapeutic state. The struggle is to re-elaborate ourselves beyond the pathologising gaze—thus the rejection of intelligibility.

Tension exists between the raucous acts of the Cynics and the instruction of Deleuze and Guattari to construct a Body without Organs, not with a sledgehammer but with a very fine file. Deleuze and Guattari are very attentive to the dangers of decomposing oneself, which, they explain, can just as easily lead to social and psychic death. The Body without Organs is thus an invitation to experiment with possible connections and flows—but to experiment piecemeal and with caution (1987, 161). Dan Goodley (2007, 153) has taken up the Body without Organs as a site for disabled people to politicise their own bodies and minds, "[w]here they [can] destabilize, perhaps at times explode, such individualised understandings of body/self/psychology/identity—in order to make connections with other bodies and entities." Likewise, becoming dysfluent and rejecting recognition is not to flip a switch (killing the organism), but to open the voice to its connections and in this way to experiment *with others* potential movements of deterritorialisation and reterritorialisation. This is how we make a "voice without organs" (Mazzei 2013).

Closely related to the rejection of recognition is, **third**, becoming imperceptible. Stuttering honestly, stuttering fiercely—stuttering from the anus—invokes a minor politic in a similar way that the Cynics invert the politics of recognition. The absolute visibility of the Cynic life is not a bid for but an open mockery of recognition. Since the Cynics were not bound by conventional principles, they could live a life "that is always in the process of becoming other, different, strange, and in this sense is always changing identity and cannot remain self-same" (Lemm 2014, 218). This scandal of otherness, Lemm continues, is in fact the *munus* or common material ground that predicates both the philosophical and political life yet is unrecognised by both. All forms of becoming-other are ultimately aimed at becoming imperceptible. The dysfluent enunciation resists intelligibility and stages becoming-other. Foucault (2003b, 134) famously claimed that "the target nowadays is not to discover what we are but to refuse what we are," and we must soberly ask whether we can refuse neoliberal subjectivisation as talking heads.

Parrhesia at its Cynic limits is a form of becoming-imperceptible. The stutter is a chop-shop that breaks the rational voice into buzzing sounds and uncanny noises, inhuman intensities and forces that unsettle the ear. This decomposition—a becoming-noise or even becoming-insect (Braidotti 2011, 100) of sound—calls the human into question but also opens new horizons of politics. "If human beings have a destiny," suggest Deleuze and Guattari (1987, 171), it is "to escape the face, to dismantle the face and facializations, to become imperceptible, to become clandestine." This is a turn from the human subject and (in)human talking-head towards what feminist theorist Hasana Sharp calls a "renaturalized" politic carefully attuned to the multiple forces that enable and constrain action. At this register, we might "see words as bodily motions caused by our mutual involvement with one another" (2011, 53). Jerked from the spell of the sociosymbolic order, disabled voices that break and repeat, stretch, and render language otherwise unintelligible are alive with forces and intensities that resist any attempt at signification and automatic connection. Sharp argues that for Deleuze and Guattari, the practice of becoming-imperceptible "target[s] not the perceptive power of nature itself but the dominant regime of perception, the social imaginary that filters, contours, and categorizes beings into intelligible entities" (177). They invite a becoming-other of sensitiveness and self.

These three Cynic themes (becoming animal, becoming unintelligible, and becoming imperceptible) are thus an escape (always partial of course) from biopolitical legibility and individuation, yet becoming other is *not* a rejection of belonging and singularity.

Schick's "Honest Speech" begins like this: "The barn owl communicates with its mates and offspring using a complex system of hissing, screeching, squawking, and facial muscle manipulation / Survival is dependent upon creating a voice so unique it can be recognized by loved ones in an instant." The barn owl does not communicate information but, instead, sounds a *refrain* that produces a territory. As Guattari writes (1995a, 15), "the simplest examples of refrains delimiting existential Territories can be found in the ethology of numerous bird species." Likewise, perhaps the dysfluent voice must be depersonalised to manifest its singularity—its connective and generative force. For disability theorist James Overboe (2012, 118), the stuttering barn owl would not represent (an identity) but express a pre-personal vitality. "We can begin to see our impairments as impersonal singularities, as generative sources—as a *thisness* of life rather than as detractors from identity." Outside the demand for recognition as filtered through market veridiction, dysfluent voices could express a singular "difference in itself."

• • •

This chapter returns to its beginning. What do the feeble-tongued have to "say" amidst our crisis of parrhesia? How might dysfluent voices speak—better: embody, live—critique in the age of info-therapeutic dominance, talking heads, trolls, and information overload? One reason I have troubled over this question is because, at least to untuned ears, only a thin line seems to separate bullshitting in the street from shitting, à la Diogenes, in the street. What do we do with the fact that listeners hungry for sound bites might not be able to differentiate the cynic from the Cynic, the toxin from the accidental refrain? Isn't shitting in the street just adding to the noise? Isn't signal and noise the only political game in town? I obsessed over these problems until I realised they expressed a vestigial "aspiration to a sort of sovereign invulnerability to the open-endedness and contingency of the future we share with others" (Markell 2003, 15). Sovereign speech is nothing but the unspinnable sound bite, the perfect word, the universal translation, each a dangerous siren.

Moreover, what distinguishes bullshit from shit is not only the pact the parrhesiastes have formed with themselves and their utterance, but more fully, a love for this world that bullshit erodes and shit nurtures.

Perhaps it is true that disability communities will always need the intelligible and respectable ally/crip who can speak the Master's tongue. Perhaps social change requires beneficent talking heads who articulate demands with quick voices commanding attention. The Master's tongue, the talking head: such authoritative devices often speak *for* the dysfluent and other demi-rhetors. To be honest, this is sometimes a relief, and from the perspective of social justice, sometimes needed. But not always. Some truths cannot be spoken nor communicated. The answer to the silencing of marginalised voices must be more than cheap talk. A smooth space is not sufficient to save us.

For McFalls and Pandolfi (2014, 185), Cynic parrhesia offers a possible escape from therapeutic governance and market veridiction. Yet this window is extremely narrow. Mobilised critically, disability can here do work. If we could feel words, with Martin, as uncanny *objects* in our mouths and the world, or with Sharp, as *bodily motions* stirred by shared affective conditions, we might awaken from an info-therapeutic slumber to not only discover the voice—and especially the dysfluent voice—as an "agentic assemblage" that is "constituted in the entanglement of *things*" (Mazzei and Jackson 2017, 1092; emphasis in original), but to recognise the power of this unruly assemblage to de-face the talking head, the currency, as a critical practice.

To stutter wildly, to stutter as a poetic, to create a vacuole of noncommunication, to fling one's shit and exit language is thus not an escape from the world. Becoming-imperceptible is a rejection, yes, of the universal ideals and projects staged by neoliberalism, but positively, it is an invitation to cultivate new existential territories and refrains in minor keys. An other, possible, life. This politic is by necessity both impure and uncertain. As Guattari (2000, 24) cautions, mental and social ecosophy never plays out deterministically, "[b] arbaric implosion cannot be entirely ruled out." Whirlpools invite dysfluency, growth, and mutation, but also toxins and cancers that pose political and existential dangers. Yet life within impure uncertainty is precisely the lesson of the Cynics—"the life philosophy of crisis" (Sloterdijk 1987, 124). The Cynics teach "moderation of expectations, adaptability, presence of mind, attention to what the moment offers" (124). Crossed lines, interruptions, and breakdowns are the exigencies and lived realities we ought to be preparing for. The Cynics offer instruction on how to navigate, live, and maybe even flourish within a dysfluent future.

Coda

Rehabilitation

I wrote this book in the age of Trump, but now release it into a different world. In November 2020, the United States shuffled into voting booths to exchange a troller-in-chief for a stutterer-in-chief. So dawned the era of rehabilitated speakers, of speech rehabilitated.

Can we note the hilarity of the "soul of the nation" (Dias 2020) being battled over by not one but *two* dysfluent white men? Trump's rhetorical style systematically hacked (apart) political discourse, but no Pericles or Obama emerged in its defense. What stumbled forth instead was a stutterer rehabilitated, a talking head who "has worked to manage his stutter [but] has also adroitly synthesized it into his public persona. It's a crucial part of his self-defined origin story" (Williams 2020). In this tired story we tell about disability, Biden "overcame" his childhood stuttering through courage and hard work and owes much of his success to surmounting this obstacle.

Of course, since stuttering can only be managed, not cured, Biden's stutter still finds opportunities to escape. And of course, Trump rarely missed an opportunity to prey on presumed weakness:

> Biden is angry. Biden is angry, everything is anger. . . . [imitating Biden's stutter]. And that's what happens when you can't get the words out, you get angry. Might happen to me one day. Can you imagine if that happened to me? Man would I be a bad guy. I would be the meanest man in history. (Zoellner 2020)

This is a telling admission by the forty-fifth US president. More interesting than the projection about his own dysfluent speech and psychological state are the series of connections he draws between blocked speech, impotence, and destructive affect. Trump here expresses yet also rewrites Brown's Paradox using an disablist trope about stuttering, where speech blocked within the body corresponds with a pathological self, festered with anger against one's own impotence and the world. At this register, individual pathology serves as a proxy for the machineries of neoliberalism that block—or better, enmesh—what we really want to say and what we really want to do and thereby incite public feelings of impotence and rage (for many on the Right, the most immediate danger is state regulation of "free speech").

But if, for some in an uncertain world, stuttering functions as a disablist metaphor for political impotence and related affect, it has become for others a site to invest in and renew political hope. It matters that Biden is *rehabilitated*-stutterer-in-chief, for, as Roshaya Rodness (2021) writes, "[his] well-publicized efforts to speak with and overcome a stutter have operated as an extended metaphor for the restoration of democracy that has now become his task in the aftermath of the political abuses under Donald Trump." Can speech be rehabilitated? Can it be trusted once again? Can the impediments to political discourse be overcome? After four years of Trump dragging discourse through the mud, we want to believe that speech can be rehabilitated in our time of need. Biden's personal narrative of overcoming is a vehicle for this desperate hope.

Inaugurations are moments of nation-building, of defining and forgetting in equal measure. The era of rehabilitated speakers and speech rehabilitated began on January 20, 2021 when the young poet laureate Amanda Gorman took the stage to read her inaugural poem "The Hill We Climb." Like Biden, Gorman had a childhood speech impediment that she has managed, yet not managed to erase. But very *unlike* Biden, Gorman is a young, Black poet and activist, a figure of the future, a far better vehicle for wounded political hope. I agree with Rodness (2021) that "[a]s we breathe new breath into democracy through poetry, representation, and marginalized voices, let us embrace renewed metaphors as well, ones divested of the damaging and ableist expectation to speak well by overcoming the intricacies of our individual voices." But at the same time, let us also remember the active power of forgetting. Let us remember that someone like Trump is merely a symptom, not a cause, of cheap talk. If we, the priesthood, are the vehicles of cheap talk, let us be ever-wary of the rebaptized word.

Notes

Introduction

1. Lazzarato (2014) and Berardi (2004) both use the term "semiocapitalism," which I prefer since it designates the integration of *part-signs* into the wheels of capitalist accumulation. The concept of "information," as I explain in chapter 2, is a technical term that doesn't fully encompass the operations of contemporary neoliberal capitalism. Nevertheless, I find *info-capitalism* useful insofar as it references the familiar concept of "information societies" and offers an accessible point that can be complexified along the way.

Chapter One

1. Much of the research on stuttering involves male participants, since stuttering occurs in a ratio of four males to every female. This is a continued source of epistemic injustice for stutterers of other genders.

2. Some (e.g., Murray 2008; Pinchevski 2011) have suggested that Bartleby is autistic, which is both an anachronistic and controversial reading.

3. For Hannah Arendt (1998), virtuosity characterises political action that cannot occur within work or labour but only outside the realm of necessity—that is, politics. Yet through the figure of the virtuoso, Virno challenges Arendt's distinction between politics and labour and suggests that labour within cognitive capitalism has increasingly taken on virtuosic characteristics traditionally belonging to the political: occurring in the midst of others, revealing one's singularity, and marked by contingency and natality. In other words, virtuosic labour is not simply interaction but the very type of interaction Arendt claims is possible only in the political sphere.

4. "I was in IT at the beginning when it was an isolated job," relays one stutterer to Butler, "But the job changed, it was more about customers and selling . . . all talk and less ability. Obviously I didn't fit his new regime and [my manager] made it obvious he wanted me out. He said that customers didn't like talking to me and that the other guys were having to work harder to make up for me" (Butler 2014, 726).

5. In both instrumentalised and affective modes of communicative labour, the voice of the workplace virtuoso is shaped by social norms such as (among others) ability and gender. Such norms constitute the subject's very capacity to speak; they are the voice's opening into the world through which the voice might appear. With regard to norms of ability, I argued above that the fulfilment of a virtuosic performance depends on the performance of aesthetic norms that are coded by compulsory able-bodiedness. The fluent virtuoso cultivates rather than blocks the flow of positive affect. But we might also consider the temporal context and performance of the virtuoso. Paterson (2012, 169) suggests that "[a] person with speech impairment 'dys-appears' because there is 'no slack' when negotiating the choreography of everyday life. One must keep 'in time' and 'in step' with the tempo of communication because slowness is the embodiment of failure and 'deficiency.'" One distinction of post-Fordist labour, the story goes, is that unlike its industrialised predecessor that standardised time within linear frames, post-Fordist labour is flexible. But the myth of temporal "slack" in the workplace and everyday life disappears immediately from the perspective of the dysfluent. The dysfluent body resists demands of temporal flexibility and thus falls out of time; the virtuoso, on the other hand, keeps "in step" within conversations. This temporal synchronisation is beneficial in the workplace, argues Butler, as research suggests it produces a greater connection with an audience, maximises identification and belonging, and increases interactional richness (721).

6. Parts of the research for this section are derived from Joshua St. Pierre and Charis St. Pierre, "Governing the Voice: A Critical History of Speech-Language Pathology," *Foucault Studies* 24 (2018): 151–84.

7. Historians such as Angela G. Ray (2005) link the rise of an oral culture organised around lyceums and Chautauqua assemblies with nation-building and the establishment of bourgeois values. Both lyceums and Chautauquas were a type of adult education movement in the nineteenth-century United States that gave people the opportunity to hear debates and lectures. Highly popular, these assemblies of performers and lecturers provided entertainment to communities.

8. Dr. Benjamin Rush was the surgeon general of Washington's army and considered by Ladelle McWhorter (2009, 102–10) to be the father of modern biopolitics.

9. Cf. St. Pierre and St. Pierre (2018, 168): "Twentieth-century speech correctionists regularly belittled elocutionists as 'quacks and charlatans' who employed archaic methods such as breathing exercises, rhythmic exercises, and vocal drills to 'fix' speech defectives for a fee. Yet while SLPs decried these practices as quackery, they continued to wield them by divorcing in growing measure their etiological from their disciplinary functions."

10. Practices to correct speech were of course not invented in the nineteenth century; stuttering, for instance, is a phenomenon that has long puzzled physicians and orators, and elocution is just one in a long line of efforts to discipline the tongue. What matters as much as the concrete practices is how they are circulated within the social field and utilised in specific ways for specific, political ends.

11. Consider Ira Wile, the commissioner of education in New York City, who in 1916 presented a paper entitled "The Economic Value of Speech Correction" to the National Education Association. Wile argued that speech defects threaten both individual and societal welfare (584). Not only is the speech defect burdensome and costly within the classroom, but "the economic cost of speech defects is registered in the limitations of occupations that are available for individuals who have speech deficiencies" (584). Wile, like many others in his time, points out employers' reticence to hire individuals with speech defects, including for jobs that required minimal speaking. In response to these concerns, speech must be rendered an object of biopolitical discourse that can in turn be governed according to the needs of a society ever more reliant on linguistic operations.

12. It is important to note that attempts to cure stuttering have returned with fervour (cf. Pittalwala 2020).

Chapter Two

1. Websites such as "Stutterbox" (https://www.stutterbox.co.uk/) and mobile apps now emulate this technology.

2. In bed is precisely where life and capitalism coexist for Paul Precardio (2013, 34), who labels contemporary capitalism a "pharmacopornographic regime."

3. Societies of control connect bodies of many sorts into global circuits of information—this is a basic operation of their power. The good worker is the good terminal: available to connect flows, often via a mobile phone, anywhere and at any time, such that value turns on interfaceability: the ability to intercommunicate with other components in an assemblage according to operational parameters. If we can forgive their outdated language, Deleuze and Guattari (1987, 570) are instructive: "[t]he issue is no longer to adapt, even under violence, but to localize: Where is your place? Even handicaps can be made useful, instead of being corrected or compensated for. A deaf-mute can be an essential part of a 'humans-machines' communicational system." Within an informational economy, deterritorialised bodies are semiotic cogs made useful through their localisation in communicative assemblages. The desire for cheap information opens up newfound possibilities if one is disabled (in a limited variety of ways) to find employment as a component part in semiotic systems.

4. We can note also that Deleuze and Guattari draw a distinction (adapted from Hjelmslev's semiotics) between the plane of content and the plane of expression. The content-plane, what Deleuze and Guattari (1987, 88) also term the "machinic assemblage of bodies," refers to the universe of corporeal bodies; expression, or the "collective assemblage of enunciation" (88), refers on the other hand to both signifier and signified—to the entire regime of the symbolic. Consider paralympic basketball. On the content-plane we find in the relations between muscles, wheelchairs, friction, gravity, and rubber, the potential of material bodies to intermingle/react and thus produce distinctly *corporeal* transformations (hardened or degraded muscles, broken wheelchairs, etc.). On the expression-plane are the callouts that

make a play, the rules that structure basketball, the regulations against doping, and the classification system that ranks the capacities of disabled athletes. The planes of content and expression interact in complex ways yet are nevertheless autonomous, operating with their own set of rules. As Eugene Holland (2013, 37) explains, these planes coexist in a relation of "reciprocal presupposition" or mutual continuativeness. The relation between content and expression thus never collapses into either gross materialism or linguistic idealism.

The machines that produce fluency do not operate exclusively on the plane of expression—the management of language and identities. To understand the production of cheap talk, we must further consider the material register of bodies (and their logics and entanglements) through which information is made to flow. This implies then that fluency machines, like all abstract machines, operate as relays between content and expression.

5. The presumption that interpersonal verbal communication is primary, Jonathan Sterne (2003, 21) argues, predetermines the history of sound from the start. "Treating face-to face communication as primary also predetermines the history of sound reproduction before we even tell the story. If interpersonal interaction is the presumptively primary or 'authentic' mode of communication, then sound reproduction is doomed to denigration as inauthentic, disorienting, and possibly even dangerous by virtue of its 'decontextualizing' sound from its 'proper' interpersonal context."

6. This logic of flattening also manifests within techniques of speech correction. Notes Richter (2020, 106): "[T]he category of speech disability becomes depoliticized precisely because its instability is primed for misunderstanding, especially by simplistic psychoanalytic, behaviorist, and neo-behaviorist analyses that all tend to reduce it to emotion, or by simplistic behaviorism that sees it as an outgrowth of failed nurturing."

7. Josephine Hoegaerts (2013, 19) argues that at the close of the nineteenth century, the human body was imagined as a nerve-system akin to a telephone exchange. The brain sent information through the nerves to the muscles. What the stutterer accordingly lacked was not willpower, but a line without interference.

8. Perhaps one reason is that stuttering exists in a liminal state between ablebodiedness and disability (St. Pierre 2012) such that many people who stutter *don't want* to identify with the disability community. While understandable in many ways (and harmful in others), this phenomenon has made collective action against ableist representations of stuttering difficult. Yet there is more at play.

Chapter Three

1. Instead of talking heads, Deleuze and Guattari might prefer the term talking *faces*, since for them, the face overcodes and delimits the human. Facialisation, the process through which the face is assembled *qua* face, rips the (rational and signifying) head from the body. "The face is produced only when the head ceases to be a part of the body, when it ceases to be coded by the body" (1987, 170). The face is

then reterritorialized on the strata of signification and subjectification where it does not express but "sets the stage" for communication: a virtual surface that reshapes the world and guides our possible relations (Rushton 2002, 234).

2. We ought, in passing, to note the asymmetry produced by stretching human capacities of communication and affectation to the inhuman limits of information machines. At the level of lived experience, the human-machine boundary (for example, prosthetic limbs) is hardly smooth but laden with friction, itches, and pain. Likewise, while information technologies are not prostheses but machinic components, the issue of mismatched interfaces is similar. Franco Berardi (2007, 81) writes that "[t]he universe of receivers—the ensemble of human brains, of real people made of flesh and fragile and sensual organs—is not formatted according to the same standards as the system of digital transmitters." Berardi skims over the ways in which humans are not just receivers but also transmitters within info-capitalism. Yet the various "pathological effects" that reside in the human-machine asymmetry are well noted: "permanent electrocution, panic, overexcitement, hypermobility, attention disorders, dyslexia, information overload, the saturation of reception circuits" (81). An info-therapeutic regime codes these structural effects as individual pathologies. This move, in turn, justifies further intervention by the high priests on fleshy organs to optimise talking heads.

3. Theorists such as Lazzarato (2015) and Harvey (2007) argue that the so-called "knowledge economy" that turns on the production/consumption of high-tech information is really a byproduct of neoliberalism and its hegemony of financial over industrial capital. Whereas industrial capital relies on labour to produce commodities and is thus embroiled in the antagonism of the capital-labour relation, financial capital is indifferent to the specific form of production and labour: "all that is relevant to them is drawing from these various forms of production and labor a surplus expressed in abstract quantities of money" (Lazzarato 2015, 141). Industrial capital has been (re)governed by financial capital since the early '70s, a hegemonic relation made possible on a global scale by expansive information technologies that process the global flows of capital, commodities, labour, and knowledge into a sufficiently mobile and deterritorialised form that financial technologies can exploit.

4. A student's knowledge stream is determined both by testing performance and career interest. However, once a student has started down one path it becomes difficult to switch due to the design of programs of study. Eugenic mechanisms lurk in such structures of curriculum that divide, for example, "theoretical" from "practical" mathematics.

5. Note that the power of a meme derives not from its truth-content but its affective resonance—its virtual power to modulate desire. For example, in the 2016 US election the alt-right weaponized and flooded social networks with the power of deterritorialised signs. With a meme, "its particular content is irrelevant. Who sent it is irrelevant. Who receives it is irrelevant" (Dean 2009, 6). Vitriolic anti-Hillary memes gained power through circulation, not understanding. One can debunk meme after meme because their continued circulation draws from a pool of "grievance politics"—specifically, in this context, cultural and racial animus.

6. This citation is curious, since Lazzarato attributes it to Deleuze but I cannot confirm its existence in the Deleuzian body of literature (though *approximations* can be found (e.g., Deleuze 2006, 85). Is this quotation a miscitation? Is it a clever commentary on the subject matter?

7. SLP reflects its humanist lineage, in which speech is connected to and expresses interiority. It remains highly "arborescent" or treelike (Deleuze and Guattari 1987) in its drive to classify, structure, and enunciate the human around a centrally organising principle—or three, in fact. Deleuze and Guattari argue that human existence is arranged and bound by three "great strata"—the *organism*, *signifying totality*, and *subjectification*: "You will be organized, you will be an organism, you will articulate your body—otherwise you're just depraved. You will be signifier and signified, interpreter and interpreted—otherwise you're just a deviant. You will be a subject, nailed down as one, a subject of the enunciation recoiled into a subject of the statement—otherwise you're just a tramp" (1987, 159). These strata mark the full human as such. Social machines, first, reduce the multiplicity of human action and desire to a singular body organised into a functional unity—the body-as-organism. They, second, require that we interpellate ourselves through a major language to, third, assume an identifiable subject position. Fluency reifies the rational organism—you will be organised by *logos*; it demands that we signify ourselves—you will be representable and represent; and it recoils the enunciation into a bounded being—you will speak not as a multiplicity but as an individual.

8. Surfaces are machined to fit through a process of what Bogard (2000) calls "marking." Similar to how a jointer peels away wood to create a level plane or shoe polish floods a fissured surface through abrasion, smoothing occurs through both extraction and deposition (270). These traces always inscribe the body. Bogard explains: "Fast and clean. Connected to all the other smooth bodies in its territory, in a smooth-running collective machine" (270). Technologies of fluency shave away undesirable speaking behaviours: tearing the event of speech from its context and web of relations. They also deposit new surfaces of (potential) contact like smooth vowels and technological devices such as the SpeechEasy. Info-therapeusis, in other words, leaves its marks when erasing marks, when it transforms dysfluent into a smooth, sterile stream. But it is important to recognise the machinic *function* of smooth speech—of fast and clean connections. Much like "the shine on a shoe 'fits' a walking-machine to a status-machine, to a commodity-machine, to a pleasure-machine, etc." (272), so does fluent speech "fit" a sound-machine to a speaking-machine, to a status-machine, to a spending-machine, to a desire-machine, to a labour-machine, etc. Fluency is a connective tissue that enables smooth contact and thus movement and relation in the social field. Fluency "fits" a subject to the speeds and rhythms of control societies; it can help smooth over misunderstanding and foster new relations.

9. Universal Design self-adheres to seven principles: (1) equitable use, (2) flexibility in use, (3) simple and intuitive use, (4) perceptible information, (5) tolerance for error, (6) low physical effort, and (7) size and space approach and use (Connell et al. 1997).

10. Google, for example, recently demonstrated voice assistant technology that could have multiple applications for dysfluent people. Google Assistant will soon be able to make reservations or book appointments with a lifelike voice that mimics the casual intonations of human speech. This artificial voice can navigate conversational turns and even language barriers. Such technologies that invite the subject into new assemblages of enunciation can forge new powers.

11. For example, Facebook allows photos to be captioned, but captions (and their facticity) are invisible unless using a screen reader. This is a form of access on demand that privatises a shared world.

Chapter Four

1. The forty-fifth US president once again springs to mind.

2. It is here worth noting that John Stuart Mill, ever the champion of liberty, was decidedly *not* in favour of the "marketplace of ideas." As Jill Gordon writes (1997, 239), "[h]is promotion of free expression does not compel Mill to recommend as a paradigm anything like a marketplace. He says that we must 'encourage' and 'countenance' the minority opinions."

3. Defined as the "turbulent woman" or "whirlwind" or "woman of masculine strength or spirit," the virago is a force of nature "that disrupts and unsettles such binary categories as masculine and feminine, point[ing] out their inadequacies, their limits, their aporias" (Honig 1993, 16).

4. In Vanessa Lemm's (2014, 210) reading, this Cynic turn is more than the simple peeling of culture from nature (*bios* to *zoe*), but a return that "reveals *zoe* as *bios*, where *zoe* is understood to be that force which gives style and form to life."

5. The parrhesiastes can also be a revolutionary figure, "one who rises within society and says: I am telling the truth, and I am telling the truth in the name of the revolution that I am going to make and that we will make together" (Foucault 2008, 70).

Bibliography

Alberta Education. 2020. *ECS to Grade 12 Guide to Education 2020–21*. Edmonton: Government of Alberta. https://open.alberta.ca/dataset/d119dba4–36cd-4e41–927b-b436fb2e75b1/resource/c9d6fa96-fbd4–433e-b193-b4281184e276/download/edc-guide-to-education-2020–2021.pdf

Arendt, Hannah. 1998. *The Human Condition*. Chicago: University of Chicago Press.

Bareilles, Sara, vocalist. 2013. "Brave." Track 1 on Sara Bareilles, *The Blessed Unrest*. Epic Records.

Beasley-Murray, Jon. 2010. *Posthegemony: Political Theory and Latin America*. Minneapolis: Minneapolis University Press.

Bell, Alexander Graham. 1908. "A Few Thoughts Concerning Eugenics." *Journal of Heredity* 1 (1): 208–14.

Bell, Alexander Graham. 1877. *Fourteenth Annual Report of the Directors and Officers of the Minnesota Institution for the Education of the Deaf and Dumb, and the Blind*. St Paul: Pioneer Press Company.

Bennett, Jane. 2001. *The Enchantment of Modern Life: Attachments, Crossings, and Ethics*. Princeton: Princeton University Press.

Bennett, Jane. 2010. *Vibrant Matter: A Political Ecology of Things*. Durham: Duke University Press.

Bennett, Jane. 2009. *The Soul at Work: From Alienation to Autonomy*. Los Angeles: Semiotext(e).

Berardi, Franco. 2011. *After the Future*. Baltimore: AK Press.

Berardi, Franco. 2007. "Schizo-Economy." Translated by Michael Goddard. *SubStance* 36 (1): 76–85. https://www.jstor.org/stable/4152854

Berlant, Lauren. 2007. "Slow Death (Sovereignty, Obesity, Lateral Agency)." *Critical Inquiry* 33 (4): 754–80. https://doi.org/10.1086/521568

BlackSpot Collective. n.d. "Fuckitall Manifesto." *Adbusters*. Accessed October 10, 2020. https://www.adbusters.org/manifesto

Bogard, William. 2000. "Smoothing Machines and the Constitution of Society." *Cultural Studies* 14 (2): 269–94. https://doi.org/10.1080/095023800334887

Bogue, Benjamin. 1912. *The Bogue Institute for Stammerers*. Cincinnati: The Procter and Collier Co.

Bonhoeffer, Dietrich. 2009. "On Stupidity." In *Letters and Papers from Prison*, edited by John W. de Gruchy, 43–44. Minneapolis: Augsburg Fortress.
Borchers, Gladys L., and Lillian R. Wagner. 1954. "Speech Education in Nineteenth-Century Schools." In *History of Speech Education in America*, edited by Karl Wallace, 277–300. New York: Appleton-Century-Crofts.
Botella, Elena. 2019. "TikTok Admits It Suppressed Videos by Disabled, Queer, and Fat Creators." *Slate,* December 4, 2019. https://slate.com/technology/2019/12/tiktok-disabled-users-videos-suppressed.html
Braidotti, Rosi. 1994. *Nomadic Subjects: Embodiment and Sexual Difference in Contemporary Feminist Theory*. New York: Columbia University Press.
Braidotti, Rosi. 2011. *Nomadic Theory: The Portable Rosi Braidotti*. New York: Columbia University Press.
Breton, Philippe. 2011. *The Culture of the Internet and the Internet as Cult: Social Fears and Religious Fantasies*. Sacramento: Litwin Books.
Brewer, Elizabeth, Cynthia L. Selfe, and Remi Yergeau. 2014. "Creating a Culture of Access in Composition Studies." *Composition Studies/Freshman English News* 42 (2): 151–54. https://www.learntechlib.org/p/153526/
Brooker, Charlie, and Konnie Huq, writers. 2011. *Black Mirror*. Series 1, episode 2, "Fifteen Million Merits." Aired December 11, 2011, on Channel 4.
Brown, Wendy. 2001. *Politics Out of History*. Princeton: Princeton University Press.
Brown, Wendy. 2015. *Undoing the Demos: Neoliberalism's Stealth Revolution*. New York: Zone Books.
Bryant, Levi R. 2014. *Onto-Cartography: An Ontology of Machines and Media*. Edinburgh: Edinburgh University Press.
Butler, Clare. 2014. "Wanted—Straight Talkers: Stammering and Aesthetic Labour." *Work, Employment and Society* 28 (5): 718–34. https://doi.org/10.1177%2F0950017013501956
Butler, Judith. 2005. *Giving an Account of Oneself*. Bronx: Fordham University Press.
Butler, Octavia E. 1993. *Parable of the Sower*. New York: Grand Central Publishing.
Campbell, Patrick. 2018. "Stammering as Weight." *Your Voice*. https://stamma.org/your-voice/stammering-weight
Campbell, Patrick, Christopher Constantino, and Sam Simpson. 2019. "Introduction." In *Stammering Pride and Prejudice*, edited by Patrick Campbell, Christopher Constantino, and Sam Simpson, xxi–xxix. Albury: J&R Press.
Carey, James. 2009. *Communication as Culture: Essays on Media and Society*. New York: Routledge.
Chrysostom, Dio. 1932. *Discourses 1–11*. New York: Harvard University Press.
Clare, Eli. 2017. *Brilliant Imperfection: Grappling with Cure*. Durham: Duke University Press.
Clearspeed. n.d. *Clearspeed*. Accessed October 17, 2020 from https://www.clearspeed.com/
Cogdell, Christina. 2004. *Eugenic Design: Streamlining America in the 1930s*. Philadelphia: University of Pennsylvania Press.
Connell, Bettye Rose, Mike Jones, Ron Mace, Jim Mueller, Abir Mullick, Elaine

Ostroff, Jon Sanford, Ed Steinfeld, Molly Story, and Gregg Vanderheiden. 1997. "The Principles of Universal Design." Version 2.0. *The Center for Universal Design*. https://projects.ncsu.edu/design/cud/about_ud/udprinciplestext.htm

Connolly, William E. 2002. *Neuropolitics: Thinking, Culture, Speed*. Minneapolis: University of Minnesota Press.

Conquergood, Dwight. 2000. "Rethinking Elocution: The Trope of the Talking Book and Other Figures of Speech." *Text and Performance Quarterly* 20 (4): 325–41. https://doi.org/10.1080/10462930009366308

Constantino, Chris. 2019. "Stutter Naked." In *Stammering Pride and Prejudice*, edited by Patrick Campbell, Christopher Constantino, and Sam Simpson, 213–23. Albury: J&R Press.

Davis, Lennard. 1996. *Enforcing Normalcy*. New York: Verso Press.

Day, Ronald E. 2001. *The Modern Invention of Information: Discourse, History, and Power*. Carbondale: Southern Illinois University Press.

Dean, Jodi. 2009. "Communication Capitalism: Circulation and the Foreclosure of Politics." *Cultural Politics* 1 (1): 51–74. https://doi.org/10.2752/174321905778054845

Deleuze, Gilles. 1997. *Essays Critical and Clinical*. Minneapolis: University of Minnesota Press.

Deleuze, Gilles. 1990. *Negotiations: 1972–1990*. New York: Columbia University Press.

Deleuze, Gilles. 1992. "Postscript on the Societies of Control." *October* 59: 3–7. https://www.jstor.org/stable/778828

Deleuze, Gilles. 2006. *Two Regimes of Madness: Texts and Interviews 1975–1995*. Cambridge, MA: Semiotext(e).

Deleuze, Gilles, and Felix Guattari. 1983. *Anti-Oedipus: Capitalism and Schizophrenia*. Minneapolis: University of Minnesota Press.

Deleuze, Gilles, and Felix Guattari. 1986. *Kafka: Toward a Minor Literature*. Translated by Dana Polan. Minneapolis: University of Minnesota Press.

Deleuze, Gilles, and Felix Guattari. 1987. *A Thousand Plateaus: Capitalism and Schizophrenia*. Edited by Brian Massumi. Minneapolis: University of Minnesota Press.

Dery, Mark. (1993) 2010. "Culture Jamming: Hacking, Slashing and Sniping in the Empire of Signs." *Mark Dery*. October 8, 2010. https://www.markdery.com/books/culture-jamming-hacking-slashing-and-sniping-in-the-empire-of-signs-2

Dias, Elizabeth. 2020. "Biden and Trump Say They're Fighting for America's 'Soul.' What Does That Mean?" *New York Times*, October 17, 2020. https://www.nytimes.com/2020/10/17/us/biden-trump-soul-nation-country.html

Dixon, Chris. 2014. *Another Politics: Talking Across Today's Transformative Movements*. Berkeley: University of California Press.

Dolmage, Jay. 2017. *Academic Ableism: Disability and Higher Education*. Ann Arbor: University of Michigan Press.

Dolmage, Jay. 2013. *Disability Rhetoric*. Syracuse: Syracuse University Press.

Dolmage, Jay. 2016. "From Steep Steps to Retrofit to Universal Design, From Collapse to Austerity: Neo-liberal Spaces of Disability." In *Disability, Space, Architecture: A Reader*, edited by Jos Boys, 102–13. New York: Routledge.

Eagle, Christopher, ed. 2013. *Literature, Speech Disorders, and Disability: Talking Normal*. New York: Routledge.

Eastman, Susan Tyler. 2006. "Designing On-Air, Print, and Budgeting in Promotion." In *Media Promotion and Marketing for Broadcasting, Cable & the Internet*, edited by Susan Tyler Eastman, Douglas A. Ferguson, Robert Klein, 127–62. Milton Park, UK: Taylor and Francis.

Elias, Jennifer. 2017. "Autistic Employees: 'We're a Good Return on Investment.'" *Silicon Valley Business Journal*, April 18, 2017. https://www.bizjournals.com/san-jose/news/2017/04/18/autism-workplace-sap-silicon-valley.html

Elliott, Carl. 2003. *Better than Well: American Medicine Meets the American Dream*. New York: W. W. Norton & Company.

Ellis, Katie, and Mike Kent. 2011. *Disability and New Media*. New York: Routledge.

Erevelles, Nirmala. 2011. *Disability and Difference in Global Contexts: Enabling a Transformative Body Politic*. New York: Palgrave Macmillan.

Eriksson, Kai. 2008. "Networks and the Philosophy of Noise." *Culture and Organization* 14 (3): 279–92. http://dx.doi.org/10.1080/14759550802270700

Faucher, Kane. 2013. *Metastasis and Metastability: A Deleuzian Approach to Information*. Rotterdam: Sense Publishers.

Feher, Michael. 2009. "Self-Appreciation; Or, the Aspirations of Human Capital." *Public Culture* 21 (1): 21–41. https://doi.org/10.1215/08992363-2008-019

Feinberg, Leslie. 1998. *Trans Liberation: Beyond Pink or Blue*. Boston: Beacon Press.

Fletcher, John Madison. 1912. "Speech Defects in Children." *American Journal of Obstetrics and Diseases of Women and Children* 65 (1): 148–49.

Forti, Simona. 2014. "Parrhesia between East and West: Foucault and Dissidence." In *The Government of Life: Foucault, Biopolitics, and Neoliberalism*, edited by Vanessa Lemm and Miguel Vatter, 187–207. New York: Fordham University Press.

Foucault, Michel. 1978. "About the Concept of the 'Dangerous Individual' in 19th-Century Legal Psychiatry." *International Journal of Law and Psychiatry* 1 (1): 1–18.

Foucault, Michel. 2008. *The Birth of Biopolitics*. New York: Picador.

Foucault, Michel. 2012. *The Courage of Truth: The Government of Self and Others II; Lectures at the Collège de France, 1983–1984*. New York: Palgrave Macmillan.

Foucault, Michel. 1995. *Discipline and Punish: The Birth of the Prison*. New York: Vintage.

Foucault, Michel. 2003a. "The Ethics of the Concern of the Self as a Practice of Freedom." In *The Essential Foucault: Selections from Essential Works of Foucault, 1954–1984*, edited by Paul Rabinow and Nikolas Rose, 25–42. New York: New Press.

Foucault, Michel. 2001. *Fearless Speech*. Edited by Joseph Pearson. Los Angeles: Semiotext(e).

Foucault, Michel. 2010. *The Government of Self and Others: Lectures at the Collège de France 1982–1983*. New York: Picador.

Foucault, Michel. 2005. *The Hermeneutics of the Subject: Lectures at the Collège de France 1981–1982*. New York: Picador.

Foucault, Michel. 1984. "On the Genealogy of Ethics: An Overview of Work in Progress." In *The Foucault Reader*, edited by Paul Rabinow, 340–72. New York: Pantheon Books.

Foucault, Michel. 1980. *Power/Knowledge: Selected Interviews and Other Writings, 1972–1977*. New York: Pantheon Books.

Foucault, Michel. 1980. "Prison Talk." In *Power/Knowledge: Selected Interviews and Other Writings, 1972–1977*, edited by Colin Gordon, 53–54. New York: Pantheon.

Foucault, Michel. 2007. *Security, Territory, Population: Lectures at the Collège de France 1977 1978*. New York: Picador.

Foucault, Michel. 2003b. "The Subject and Power." In *The Essential Foucault*, edited by Paul Rabinow and Nikolas Rose, 126–44. New York: New Press.

Frankfurt, Harry. 2005. *On Bullshit*. Princeton: Princeton University Press.

Freeman, Elizabeth. 2010. *Time Binds: Queer Temporalities, Queer Histories*. Durham: Duke University Press.

Fritsch, Kelly. 2015. "Gradations of Debility and Capacity: Biocapitalism and the Neoliberalization of Disability Relations." *Canadian Journal of Disability Studies* 4 (2): 12–48. https://doi.org/10.15353/cjds.v4i2.208

Galton, Francis. 1883. *Inquiries into Human Faculty and Its Development*. London: Macmillan. https://archive.org/details/inquiriesintohu00galtgoog/page/n42/mode/2up

Garland-Thomson, Rosemarie. 2012. "The Case for Conserving Disability." *Journal of Bioethical Inquiry* 9 (3): 339–55. https://doi.org/10.1007/s11673-012-9380-0

Garland-Thomson, Rosemarie. 1997. *Extraordinary Bodies: Figuring Physical Disability in American Culture and Literature*. New York: Columbia University Press.

Gleeson, Brendan. 1999. *Geographies of Disability*. New York: Routledge.

Gleick, James. 2012. *The Information: A History, A Theory, A Flood*. New York: Pantheon Books.

Glezos, Simon. 2021. *Speed and Micropolitics: Bodies, Minds, Perceptions in an Accelerating World*. New York: Routledge.

Goodley, Dan. 2007. "Becoming Rhizomatic Parents: Deleuze, Guattari and Disabled Babies." *Disability & Society* 22 (2): 145–60. https://doi.org/10.1080/09687590601141576

Goodley, Dan. 2014. *Dis/Ability Studies: Theorising Disablism and Ableism*. New York: Routledge.

Gordon, Jill. 1997. "John Stuart Mill and the 'Marketplace of Ideas.'" *Social Theory and Practice* 23 (2): 235–49. https://doi.org/10.5840/soctheorpract199723210

Greene, James Sonnett. 1916. "The Mission of the Speech Specialist." In *The National Education Association's Journal of Proceedings and Addresses (54th Meeting)*, 865–67. Ann Arbor: National Education Association.

Guattari, Felix. 1995a. *Chaosmosis: An Ethico-Aesthetic Paradigm*. Bloomington: Indiana University Press.

Guattari, Felix. 1996. *The Guattari Reader*. Edited by Gary Genosko. Hoboken: Blackwell.

Guattari, Felix. 1995b. "On Machines." *Complexity: Architecture / Art / Philosophy* 6: 8–12.

Guattari, Felix. 1977. *La Révolution Moléculaire*. Fonrenay-sous-Bois: Recherches.

Guattari, Felix. 2000. *The Three Ecologies*. Translated by Ian Pindar and Paul Sutton. London: Athlone Press.

Guitar, Barry. 2006. *Stuttering: An Integrated Approach to its Nature and Treatment*. 3rd ed. Baltimore: Lippincott Williams & Wilkins.

Hagood, Mack. 2019. *Hush: Media and Sonic Self-Control*. Durham: Duke University Press.

Hale, Lester L. 1954. "Dr. James Rush—Psychologist and Voice Scientist." *Quarterly Journal of Speech* in *History of Speech* 35 (4): 448–55.

Hamraie, Aimi. 2017. *Building Access: Universal Design and the Politics of Disability*. Minneapolis: University of Minnesota Press.

Hamraie, Aimi, and Kelly Fritsch. 2019. "Crip Technoscience Manifesto." *Catalyst: Feminism, Theory, Technoscience* 5 (1): 1–34. https://doi.org/10.28968/cftt.v5i1.29607

Haraway, Donna. 1990. *Simians, Cyborgs, and Women: The Reinvention of Nature*. New York: Routledge.

Hardt, Michael. 1999. "Affective Labor." *boundary 2* 26 (2): 89–100. http://www.jstor.org/stable/303793?origin=JSTOR-pdf

Harvey, David. 2007. *A Brief History of Neoliberalism*. New York: Oxford University Press.

Hayles, Katherine. 1999. *How We Became Posthuman: Virtual Bodies in Cybernetics, Literature, and Informatics*. Chicago: University of Chicago Press.

Heidegger, Martin. 1962. *Being and Time*. Translated by John Maxquarrie and Edward Robinson. Cambridge, UK: Blackwell.

Heyes, Cressida. 2007. *Self-Transformations: Foucault, Ethics, and Normalized Bodies*. New York: Oxford University Press.

Hoegaerts, Josephine. 2013. "'Is It a Habit or Is It a Disease?' The Changing Social Meaning of Stammering in Nineteenth-Century Western Europe." *Terrains & Travaux* 23: 17–37. https://doi.org/10.3917/tt.023.0017

Holland, Eugene. 2013. *Deleuze and Guattari's 'A Thousand Plateaus': A Reader's Guide*. New York: Bloomsbury.

Homer-Dixon, Thomas. 2000. *The Ingenuity Gap: How We Can Solve the Problems of the Future*. Toronto: Knopf.

Honig, Bonnie. 1993. *Political Theory and the Displacement of Politics*. Ithaca: Cornell University Press.

Huws, Ursula. 2014. *Labor in the Global Digital Economy: The Cybertariat Comes of Age*. New York: Monthly Review Press.

Jaarsma, Ada. 2020. "Critical Disability Studies and the Problem of Method." In *Trandisciplinary Feminist Research*, edited by Carol A. Taylor, Jasmine Ulmer, and Christina Huges, 16–28. New York: Routledge.

Jaarsma, Ada. 2017. *Kierkegaard After the Genome: Science, Existence, and Belief in This World*. New York: Palgrave MacMillan.

Jacoby, Sanford M. 2004. *Employing Bureaucracy: Managers, Unions, and the Transformation of Work in the 20th Century*. Mahwah, NJ: Lawrence Erlbaum Associates.

Janus Development Group. n.d. *SpeechEasy*. Accessed February 11, 2020 from https://speecheasy.com/

Kafer, Alison. 2013. *Feminist, Queer, Crip*. Bloomington: Indiana University Press.

Keller, Hellen. 1949. "Bell Laboratories Record." Helen Keller Archive. https://www.afb.org/HelenKellerArchive?a=d&d=A-HK01-02-B035-F06-009.1.20

Kurihara, Kazutaka, and Koji Tsukada. 2012. "SpeechJammer: A System Utilizing Artificial Speech Disturbance with Delayed Auditory Feedback. Extended Abstract." *arXiv* 1202.6106: 1–10. https://arxiv.org/vc/arxiv/papers/1202/1202.6106v1.pdf

Lacey, Kate 2013. *Listening Publics: The Politics and Experience of Listening in the Media Age*. New York: John Wiley and Sons.

Latour, Bruno. 2014. "Anthropology at the Time of the Anthropocene: A Personal View of What Is to Be Studied." In *The Anthropology of Sustainability: Beyond Development and Progress*, edited by Marc Brightman and Jerome Lewis, 35–49. New York: Palgrave Macmillan.

Lawlor, Leonard. 2016. *From Violence to Speaking Out: Apocalypse and Expression in Foucault, Derrida, and Deleuze*. Edinburgh: Edinburgh University Press.

Lazzarato, Maurizio. 2015. *Governing by Debt*. South Pasadena: Semiotext(e).

Lazzarato, Maurizio. 1996. "Immaterial Labour." In *Radical Thought in Italy: A Potential Politics*, edited by Paolo Virno and Michael Hardt, 132–47. Minneapolis: University of Minnesota Press.

Lazzarato, Maurizio. 2006. "The Machine." Translated by Mary O'Neill. *Transversal Texts*, October 1, 2006. http://eipcp.net/transversal/1106/lazzarato/en

Lazzarato, Maurizio. 2014. *Signs and Machines: Capitalism and the Production of Subjectivity*. Los Angeles: Semiotext(e).

Leder, Drew. 1990. *The Absent Body*. Chicago: University of Chicago Press.

Lemm, Vanessa. 2014. "The Embodiment of Truth and the Politics of Community: Foucault and the Cynics." In *The Government of Life: Foucault, Biopolitics, and Neoliberalism*, edited by Vanessa Lemm and Miguel Vatter, 208–23. New York: Fordham University Press.

Lipardi, Lisbeth. (2014). *Listening, Thinking, Being: Toward an Ethics of Attunement*. University Park: Penn State University Press.

Lugones, Maria. 1987. "Playfulness, 'World'-Travelling, and Loving Perception." *Hypatia* 2 (2): 3–19. https://doi.org/10.1111/j.1527-2001.1987.tb01062.x

Lugones, Maria. 1994. "Purity, Impurity, and Separation." *Signs* 19 (2): 458–79. https://www.jstor.org/stable/3174808

Lugones, Maria, and Elizabeth Spelman. 1983. "Have We Got a Theory for You! Feminist Theory, Cultural Imperialism and the Demand for 'the Woman's Voice.'" *Women's Studies International Forum* 6 (6): 573–81. https://doi.org/10.1016/0277-5395(83)90019-5

Lyotard, Jean-François. 1984. *The Postmodern Condition: A Report on Knowledge.* Minneapolis: University of Minnesota Press.

MacLure, Maggie. 2009. "Broken Voices, Dirty Words: On the Productive Insufficiency of Voice." In *Voice in Qualitative Inquiry: Challenging Conventional, Interpretive, and Critical Conceptions in Qualitative Research,* edited by Alecia Y. Jackson and Lisa A. Mazzei, 97–113. New York: Routledge.

Madison, James. 1865. "Letter to William T. Barry, 1822." In *Letters and Other Writings of James Madison, Volume 3,* 276–78. Philadelphia: J. B. Lippincott & Co.

Mao Zedong. 1972. *Quotations from Chairman Mao Tsetung.* Peking: Foreign Languages Press.

Marazzi, Christian. 2008. *Capital and Language: From the New Economy to the War Economy.* Los Angeles: Semiotext(e).

Markell, Patchen. 2003. *Bound by Recognition.* Princeton: Princeton University Press.

Marshall, James D. 1999. "Performativity: Lyotard and Foucault Through Searle and Austin." *Studies in Philosophy and Education* 18 (5): 309–17. https://doi.org/10.1023/A:1005272607727

Martin, Daniel. 2021. "'D-d-d-don't st-st-trike him, he st-t-t-tutters s-same as as w-we d-d-d do': Stammering Jokes, Wit, and Humor Since the 19th Century." Paper presented at the Metaphoric Stammers and Embodied Speakers: Connecting Clinical, Cultural and Creative Practice in the Area of Dysfluency Conference. Online, April 2021.

Martin, Daniel. 2020. "Speech: Dysfluent Temporalities in the Long Nineteenth Century." In *A Cultural History of Disability in the Long Nineteenth Century (A Cultural History of Disability, Volume 5),* edited by Joyce L. Huff and Martha Stoddard Holmes, 113–28. New York: Bloomsbury Academic.

Martin, Daniel. 2016. "Stuttering from the Anus." *Canadian Journal of Disability Studies* 5 (3): 114–34. https://doi.org/10.15353/cjds.v5i3.299

Marx, Karl. 1976. *Capital, Volume 1.* Translated by Ben Fowkes. London: Penguin Classics.

Marx, Karl. 1973. *Grundrisse: Foundations of the Critique of Political Economy.* New York: Penguin Books.

Maynes, Charles. 2019. "The Trolls Are Winning, Says Russian Troll Hunter." *The World,* March 13, 2019. https://www.pri.org/stories/2019-03-13/trolls-are-winning-says-russian-troll-hunter

Mazzei, Lisa A. 2013. "A Voice Without Organs: Interviewing in Posthumanist Research." *International Journal of Qualitative Studies in Education* 26 (6): 732–40. https://doi.org/10.1080/09518398.2013.788761

Mazzei, Lisa A., and Alecia Y. Jackson. 2017. "Voice in the Agentic Assemblage." *Educational Philosophy and Theory* 49 (11): 1090–98. https://doi.org/10.1080/00131857.2016.1159176

McDonald, Dennis J. 1916. "Speech Improvement." In *The National Education Association's Journal of Proceedings and Addresses (54th Meeting),* 862–65. Ann Arbor: National Education Association.

McFalls, Laurence, and Mariella Pandolfi. 2014. "Parrhesia and Therapeusis: Foucault on and in the World of Contemporary Neoliberalism." In *Foucault Now: Current Perspective in Foucault Studies*, edited by James D. Faubion, 168–87. Malden: Polity.

McGuire, Anne, and Kelly Fritsch. 2019. "Fashioning the 'Normal' Body." In *Power and Everyday Practices*, edited by Deborah Brock, Aryn Martin, Rebecca Raby, and Mark Thomas, 79–99. Toronto: University of Toronto Press.

McRuer, Robert. 2012. "Cripping Queer Politics, or the Dangers of Neoliberalism." *Scholar & Feminist Online* 10 (1–2): 1–2. http://sfonline.barnard.edu/a-new-queer-agenda/cripping-queer-politics-or-the-dangers-of-neoliberalism/

McRuer, Robert. 2006. *Crip Theory: Cultural Signs of Queerness and Disability*. New York: New York University Press.

McRuer, Robert. 2018. *Crip Times: Disability, Globalization, and Resistance*. New York: New York University Press.

McRuer, Robert, and Anna Mollow. 2012. *Sex and Disability*. Durham: Duke University Press.

McWhorter, Ladelle. 2009. *Racism and Sexual Oppression in Anglo-America: A Genealogy*. Bloomington: Indiana University Press.

Melville, Herman. (1853) 1995. *Bartleby, The Scrivener: A Story of Wall-Street*. Minneapolis: Indulgence Press.

Mills, Mara. 2011. "On Disability and Cybernetics: Helen Keller, Norbert Wiener, and the Hearing Glove." *Differences* 22 (2–3): 74–111. https://doi.org/10.1215/10407391-1428852

Mitchell, David, and Sharon Snyder. 2010. "Disability as Multitude: Re-working Non-Productive Labor Power." *Journal of Literary & Cultural Disability Studies* 4 (2): 179–93. https://doi.org/10.1007/978-981-287-532-7_279-1

Moore, Jason W. 2015. *Capitalism in the Web of Life: Ecology and the Accumulation of Capital*. New York: Verso.

Moten, Fred and Stefano Harney. 2013. *The Undercommons: Fugitive Planning & Black Study*. New York: Minor Compositions.

Mumford, Lewis. 1934. *Technics and Civilization*. New York: Harcourt, Brace and Company.

Murray, Stuart. 2008. *Representing Autism: Culture, Narrative, Fascination*. Liverpool: Liverpool University Press.

Nichols, Marie Hochmuth, and Richard Murphy. 1954. "Rhetorical and Elocutionary Training in Nineteenth-Century Colleges." In *History of Speech Education In America*, edited by Karl Wallace, 153–77. New York: Appleton-Century-Crofts.

Nietzsche, Friedrich. 2006. "Homer's Contest." In *'On the Genealogy of Morality' and Other Writings*, edited by Keith Ansell-Pearson, 174–82. Cambridge: Cambridge University Press.

Nimmo, Dan, and James Combs. 1992. *The Political Pundits*. New York: Praeger.

Noll, Mark A. 1994. *The Scandal of the Evangelical Mind*. Grand Rapids: InterVarsity Press.

Olkowski, Dorothea. 1999. *Gilles Deleuze and the Ruin of Representation*. Berkeley: University of California Press.

Orwell, George. 2008. *1984*. New York: Penguin Books.

O'Toole, Corbett. 2015. *Fading Scars: My Queer Disability History*. Fort Worth: Autonomous Press.

Overboe, James. 2012. "Theory, Impairment, and Impersonal Singularities: Deleuze, Guattari and Agamben." In *Disability and Social Theory: New Developments and Directions*, edited by Dan Goodley, Bill Hughes, and Lennard Davis, 112–26. New York: Palgrave.

Padden, Carol. 2015. "Communication." In *Keywords for Disability Studies*, edited by Rachel Adams, Benjamin Reiss, and David Serlin, 43–45. New York: New York University Press.

Paterson, Kevin. 2012. "It's About Time! Understanding the Experience of Speech Impairment." In *Routledge Handbook of Disability Studies*, edited by Alan Roulstone and Carol Thomas Nick Watson, 165–77. New York: Routledge.

Paul, Christopher, and Miriam Matthews. 2016. "The Russian 'Firehose of Falsehood' Propaganda Model: Why It Might Work and Options to Counter It." *RAND Corporation*. https://www.rand.org/pubs/perspectives/PE198.html

Peters, John Durham. 1989. "Locke, the Individual, and the Origin of Communication." *Quarterly Journal of Speech* 75 (4): 387–99. https://doi.org/10.1080/00335638909383886

Peters, John Durham. 1999. *Speaking into the Air: A History of the Idea of Communication*. Chicago: University of Chicago Press.

Phillips, Whitney. 2015. *This Is Why We Can't Have Nice Things: Mapping the Relationship Between Online Trolling and Mainstream Culture*. Cambridge: MIT Press.

Pinchevski, Amit. 2011. "Bartleby's Autism: Wandering Along Incommunicability." *Cultural Critique* 78 (2): 27–59. https://doi.org/10.5749/culturalcritique.78.2011.0027

Pindar, Ian, and Paul Sutton. 2000. Translator's introduction to *The Three Ecologies*, by Felix Guattari, 1–11. London: Athlone Press.

Pitawalla, Iqbal. 2020. "School of Medicine to Serve as Lead Site for Clinical Trial on Stuttering." *UC Riverside News*, December 15, 2020. https://news.ucr.edu/articles/2020/12/15/school-medicine-serve-lead-site-clinical-trial-stuttering

Plato. 1994. *Gorgias*. Translated by Robin Waterfield. New York: Oxford University Press.

Preciado, Paul B. 2013. *Testo Junkie: Sex, Drugs, and Biopolitics in the Pharmacopornographic Era*. Translated by Bruce Benderson. New York: Feminist Press.

Preston, Katherine. 2014. "Honest Speech: How Do the Ways We Modify Our Voices Affect Our Identity?" *Psychology Today*, November 13, 2014. https://www.psychologytoday.com/ca/blog/out-it/201411/honest-speech

Puar, Jasbir K. 2013. "The Cost of Getting Better: Ability and Debility." In *The Disability Studies Reader*, edited by Lennard J. Davis, 177–84. New York: Routledge.

Ray, Angela G. 2005. *The Lyceum and Public Culture in the Nineteenth-Century United States*. East Lansing: Michigan State University Press.

Read, Jason. 2003. *The Micro-Politics of Capital: Marx and the Prehistory of the Present*. New York: State University of New York Press.

Reddy, Michael J. 1979. "The Conduit Metaphor: A Case of Frame Conflict in Our Language About Language." In *Metaphor and Thought*, edited by Andrew Ortony, 284–310. Cambridge: Cambridge University Press.

Richter, Zara. 2020. "Speech Disability's Awkward Late Modernity: A Multimodal Historical Approach." In *A Cultural History of Disability in the Modern Age*. Volume 6, *A Cultural History of Disability*, edited by David T. Mitchell and Sharon L. Snyder, 95–109. New York: Bloomsbury Academic.

Rodness, Roshaya. 2021. "From Biden to 'Bridgerton,' How Our Stuttering Heroes Bring a Restoration of Democracy." *Salon*, February 28, 2021. https://www.salon.com/2021/02/28/joe-biden-bridgerton-stutter-democracy-amanda-gorman/

Rosa, Hartmut. 2010. *Alienation and Acceleration: Toward a Critical Theory of Late-Modern Temporality*. Copenhagen: Nordic Summer University Press.

Rose, Nikolas. 2007. *The Politics of Life Itself: Biomedicine, Power, and Subjectivity in the Twenty-First Century*. Princeton: Princeton University Press.

Rush, James. 1827. *The Philosophy of the Human Voice*. Philadelphia: J. Maxwell.

Rushton, Richard. 2002. "What Can a Face Do? On Deleuze and Faces." *Cultural Critique* 51: 219–37. https://www.jstor.org/stable/1354641

Russell, Marta, and Ravi Malhotra. 2002. "Capitalism and Disability." *Socialist Register* 38: 211–28. https://socialistregister.com/index.php/srv/article/view/5784

Sansome, Simon. 2019. "Disability Is Not Good for Facebook Says: 'Facebook.'" *Ability Access*, April 8, 2019. https://abilityaccess.blog/2019/04/08/breaking-news-disability-is-not-good-for-facebook-says-facebook/

Sartre, Jean Paul. 1948. *Anti-Semite and Jew*. New York: Schocken Books.

Savat, David, and Tauel Harper. 2016. *Media After Deleuze*. New York: Bloomsbury Academic.

Scheuer, Jeffrey. 2001. *The Sound Bite Society: How Television Helps the Right and Hurts the Left*. New York: Routledge.

Schick, Erin. 2014. "Honest Speech." Button Poetry, August 21, 2014. YouTube Video, 3:19. https://www.youtube.com/watch?v=j8XOyY54-Ew

Schweik, Susan. 2009. *The Ugly Laws: Disability in Public*. New York: New York University Press.

Scripture, Edward Wheeler. 1912. *Stuttering and Lisping*. New York: Macmillan Company.

Shannon, Claude, and Warren Weaver. 1963. *The Mathematical Theory of Communication*. Champaign: University of Illinois Press.

Sharma, Sarah. 2020. "A Manifesto for the Broken Machine." *Camera Obscura* 35 (2): 170–79. https://doi.org/10.1215/02705346-8359652

Sharma, Sarah. 2014. *In the Meantime: Temporality and Cultural Politics*. Durham: Duke University Press.

Sharp, Hasana. 2011. *Spinoza and the Politics of Renaturalization*. Chicago: University of Chicago Press.

Sheridan, Thomas. 1762. *A Course of Lectures on Elocution*. London: W. Strahan.

Schildrick, Margrit. 1997. *Leaky Bodies and Boundaries: Feminism, Postmodernism and (Bio)ethics*. New York: Routledge.

Shotwell, Alexis. 2016. *Against Purity: Living Ethically in Compromised Times*. Minneapolis: University of Minnesota Press.
Simmons, Kylie. 2016. "I Was Detained at an Airport Because of My Stutter." *HerCampus* October 11, 2016. https://www.hercampus.com/school/k-college/i-was-detained-airport-because-my-stutter-0
Simon, Clarence. 1954. "Development of Education in Speech and Hearing to 1920." In *History of Speech Education in America*, edited by Karl Wallace, 389–421. New York: Appleton-Century-Crofts.
Simplican, Stacy. 2015. *The Capacity Contract: Intellectual Disability and the Question of Citizenship*. Minneapolis: University of Minnesota Press.
Sloterdijk, Peter. 1987. *Critique of Cynical Reason*. Minneapolis: University of Minnesota Press.
Smith, Daniel, and John Protevi. 2018. "Gilles Deleuze." In *The Stanford Encyclopedia of Philosophy*, edited by Edward N. Zalta. https://plato.stanford.edu/archives/spr2020/entries/deleuze/
Spinoza. 1994. *A Spinoza Reader: Ethics and Other Works*. Edited and translated by Edwin Curley. Princeton: Princeton University Press.
St. Pierre, Joshua. 2012. "The Construction of the Disabled Speaker: Locating Stuttering in Disability Studies." *Canadian Journal of Disability Studies* 1 (3): 1–21. https://doi.org/10.15353/cjds.v1i3.54
St. Pierre, Joshua. 2015. "Distending Straight-Masculine Time: A Phenomenology of the Disabled Speaking Body." *Hypatia* 30 (1): 49–65. https://doi.org/10.1111/hypa.12128
St. Pierre, Joshua, and Charis St. Pierre. 2018. "Governing the Voice: A Critical History of Speech-Language Pathology." *Foucault Studies* 24: 151–84. https://doi.org/10.22439/fs.v0i24.5530
Starkweather, C. Woodruff. 1987. *Fluency and Stuttering*. Englewood Cliffs: Prentice-Hall.
Sterne, Jonathan. 2003. *The Audible Past: Cultural Origins of Sound Reproduction*. Durham: Duke University Press.
Taylor, Sunny. 2004. "The Right Not to Work: Power and Disability." *Monthly Review: An Independent Magazine*, March 1, 2004. https://monthlyreview.org/2004/03/01/the-right-not-to-work-power-and-disability/
Terranova, Tiziana. 2004. *Network Culture: Politics for the Information Age*. Ann Arbor: Pluto Press.
Tomlinson, John. 2007. *The Culture of Speed: The Coming of Immediacy*. Los Angeles: Sage Publications.
Tremain, Shelley. 2017. *Foucault and Feminist Philosophy of Disability*. Ann Arbor: University of Michigan Press.
Tremain, Shelley. 2001. "On the Government of Disability." *Social Theory and Practice* 24 (4): 617–36. https://doi.org/10.5840/soctheorpract200127432
Tsing, Anna Lowenhaupt. 2015. *The Mushroom at the End of the World: On the Possibility of Life in Capitalist Ruins*. Princeton: Princeton University Press.
U.S. Customs and Border Patrol. 2018. "On a Typical Day in Fiscal Year 2017,

CBP . . ." *Department of Homeland Security*. Updated February 13, 2018. https://www.cbp.gov/newsroom/stats/typical-day-fy2017

U.S. House Committee on Energy and Commerce. 2020. Testimony by Tim Kendall. Included in *Mainstreaming Extremism: Social Media's Role in Radicalizing America*. 116th Congress. September 24, 2020. https://docs.house.gov/meetings/IF/IF17/20200924/111041/HHRG-116-IF17-Wstate-KendallT-20200924.pdf

Usborne, Simon. 2017. "The Expert Whose Children Gatecrashed His TV Interview: 'I Thought I'd Blown It in Front of the Whole World.'" *The Guardian*, December 20, 2017. https://www.theguardian.com/media/2017/dec/20/robert-kelly-south-korea-bbc-kids-gatecrash-viral-storm

Van Riper, Charles. 1939. *Speech Correction: Principles and Methods*. New York: Prentice Hall.

Virilio, Paul. 1999. *The Information Bomb*. New York: Verso.

Virilio, Paul. 1997. *Open Sky*. New York: Verso.

Virilio, Paul, and Sylvere Lotringer. 2002. *Crepuscular Dawn*. Translated by Mike Taormina. Los Angeles: Semiotext(e).

Virno, Paolo. 2004. *Grammar of the Multitude*. South Pasadena: Semiotext(e).

Virno, Paolo. 2001. "Labor and Language." In *Lexicon of Postfordism*, edited by Adelino Zanini and Ubaldo Fadini. Translated by Arianna Bove. Milan: Feltrinelli. http://www.generation-online.org/t/labourlanguage.htm

Wiener, Anna. 2020. *Uncanny Valley: A Memoir*. New York: MCD.

Wiener, Norbert. 1950. *The Human Use of Human Beings: Cybernetics and Society*. Boston: Houghton Mifflin.

Wiener, Norbert. 1949. "Sound Communication with the Deaf." *Philosophy of Science* 16 (3): 260–62. https://www.jstor.org/stable/185520

Wile, Ira S. 1916. "The Economic Value of Speech Correction." In *The National Education Association's Journal of Proceedings and Addresses (54th Meeting)*, 875–77. Ann Arbor: National Education Association.

Williams, Mary Elizabeth. 2020. "Why Joe Biden's Stutter Is a Gift to America." *Salon*, December 26, 2020. https://www.salon.com/2020/12/26/why-joe-bidens-stutter-is-a-gift-to-america/

Wolf, Michelle, host. 2018. *The Break*. Season 1, episode 3, "Bad Opinions." Aired June 10, 2018, on Netflix.

World Health Organization. 2019. "Sanitation: Key Facts." *World Health Organization*. June 14, 2019. https://www.who.int/news-room/fact-sheets/detail/sanitation

Yergeau, Remi. 2018. *Authoring Autism: On Rhetoric and Neurological Queerness*. Durham: Duke University Press.

Young, Molly. 2020. "Garbage Language: Why Do Corporations Speak the Way They Do?" *Vulture* (Feb. 20). https://www.vulture.com/2020/02/spread-of-corporate-speak.html

Zoellner, Danielle. 2020. "Trump Slurs Through Speech as He Mocks Joe Biden's Stutter." *Independent*, February 21, 2020. https://www.independent.co.uk/video/

trump-speech-today-slur-joe-biden-stutter-maga-rally-las-vegas-a9352036.html
Zuckerberg, Mark. 2010. "Is Connectivity a Human Right?" *Facebook*. https://www.facebook.com/isconnectivityahumanright

Index

Printed and bound by CPI Group (UK) Ltd, Croydon, CR0 4YY

20/08/2025

14722219-0005